Strength Training
For Muscle Development

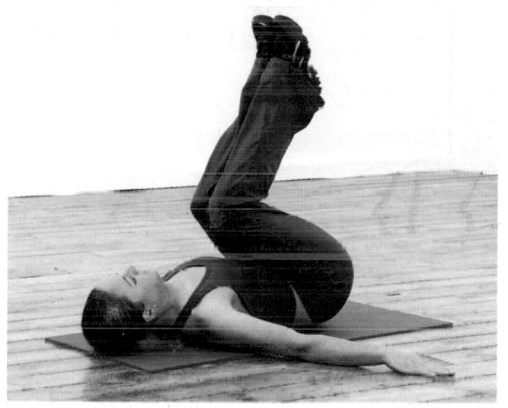

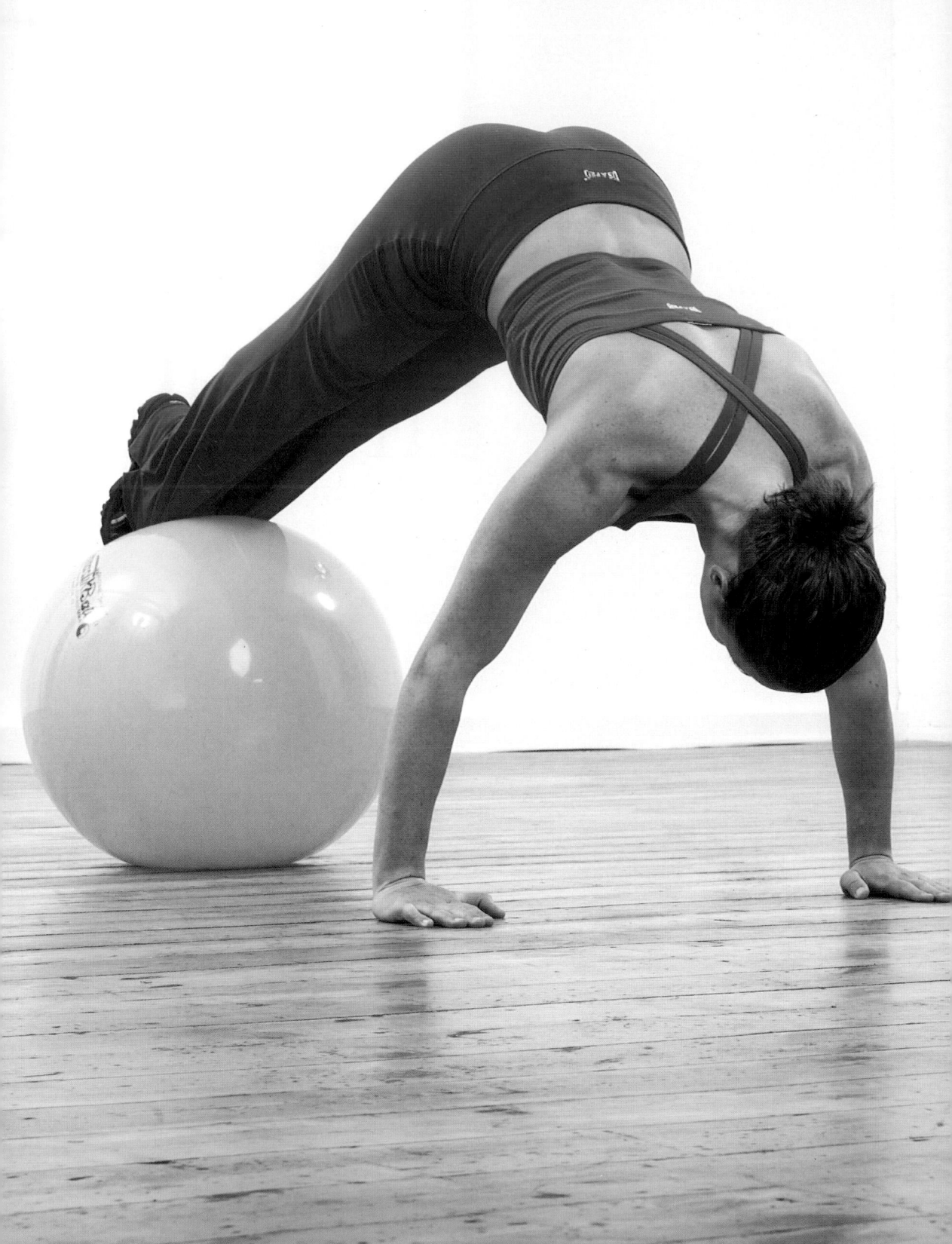

Strength Training
For Muscle Development

A STEP-BY-STEP GUIDE

IMPROVE YOUR STRENGTH

20-MINUTE WORKOUTS

Mark Hatfield

BARNES & NOBLE BOOKS

NEW YORK

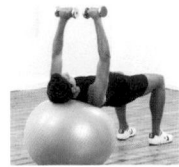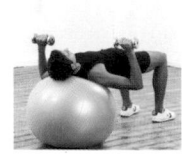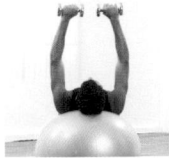

This edition published by Barnes and Noble Inc.,
by arrangement with PRC Publishing

2005 Barnes and Noble Books

M 10 9 8 7 6 5 4 3 2

ISBN 0-7607-6474-3

Produced by PRC Publishing
The Chrysalis Building
Bramley Road, London W10 6SP

An imprint of **Chrysalis** Books Group plc

Printed in China

Contents

Introduction

You have picked up a strength-training book. You just might be about to achieve a better quality of life. A tall order you may think, but most people will find some benefit from reading this book and applying the knowledge gained.

If you have never considered using weights for exercise before, or have always been put off by those in the gym who look like they know what they are doing, read on. You will find a wealth of information you can use every day to boost your confidence. If you have been exercising for some time, but for whatever reason the use of weights has never appealed, find out what you have been missing! It may be the kick that you have been looking for to spur you on to that next stage in your quest for health and fitness. Or if you have been doing some form of resistance training and you need some new material to stave off the boredom, there may be something here you have never thought of before.

And the best part? Well, how about all of this and being able to do it from the comfort of your own home in about twenty minutes? Minimal equipment. Minimal cost. Maximum benefit.

What is resistance training?

For our purposes, there is no need to worry about the difference between wieght lifting and weight training. Both approaches share one common principle, the use of some form of resistance, or weight. You are lifting a resistance through a range of movement. Even conditioning classes use some sort of strength training principle. So you don't have to have, or want to develop, huge muscles or heave huge weights over your head to take part in resistance training. Unless your goal is really significant muscle mass: in which case, heavy weights are necessary.

Because we are using several different types of weights and resistance providers (see Equipment, page 10) and not all of them strictly weights, we will refer to the type of training as Resistance Training. This means any movement where your muscle is having a force applied that it has to move against to overcome.

What is the effect?

Let us first get rid of one resistance training demon and tell you what it won't do. Nobody is hypersensitive to lifting: just because you are doing it in a controlled and focussed manner, you will not suddenly develop huge muscles, a questionable tan, and an unnerving desire to wear the smallest, most brightly colored beachwear available. The guys and girls who do have physiques like this will spend many, many, *many* hours in the gym, lifting big weights, eating a massive amount, and in some cases, taking banned substances to further develop their musculature. If you can look at that list of requirements and tick no to all of them, then this will not happen to you by following the exercises and the workouts here.

What you will get from this book is an easy-to-follow guide on how to use resistance. You will become stronger, your body will become more toned, you will reduce your body fat, boost your metabolism, increase your bone density, and improve your own self-esteem, in the knowledge that you, and only you, are doing something to improve yourself. The last benefit is priceless on its own.

How many times during the day do you wish life was a little bit easier? If you are stronger then all those chores, at home or work, that require effort, will all start to feel so much easier. Whether it's playing with the kids, carrying the groceries, or changing a wheel, imagine how it would feel when one day these tasks becamse nowhere near as strenuous.

Without some sort of stimulus you get bored and boredom feeds on itself: the less input, the less you are interested. Similarly, your muscles are lazy! They will only do what is asked of them, and no more. So if you do not use your muscles, they won't improve. You have to give them something to do. If you lead a sedentary lifestyle, sit down in an office all day, and drive to work and back, then your muscles are not being challenged at all. So they adapt to this stimulus and become softer and smaller because they can still do what you ask of them. It is only when you ask more of them that they will fail. This is why, with resistance training, you must

make small changes as you go along. Start small and build up to give your muscles that constant challenge. If you don't, they will become lazy again until you give them something new.

What if you could burn more calories just sitting on your butt and doing nothing? It is possible, if you can change your base metabolism—the number of calories that you need each day to function, simply to stay alive. This is the energy you need to breathe, maintain body temperature, and digest

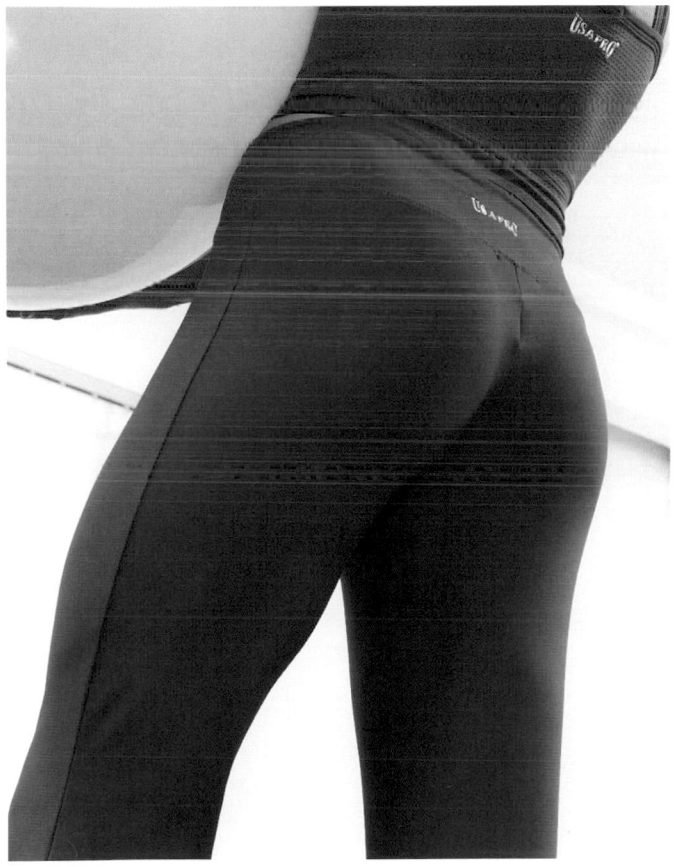

food. The best way to boost your metabolism so that you need more calories for these functions is to increase your lean muscle mass—resistance training does just that.

Muscles are the main metabolically active tissue in the body. When you work your muscles against a resistance, over time the muscle fibers become denser and increase in size. The more muscle you have, the more calories you burn.

For guys this is easier as they are naturally able to build more muscle than women. So women should not be scared to push and lift the heavier weights. They won't turn into muscle-bound monsters!

Right down to the bone

One element of your physique that you probably do not worry about too much is your bones. Over time your skeleton can become brittle. Osteoporosis is a deterioration of the bone tissue that leads to the bone becoming fragile, so if you take a fall, your chances of a

fracture are greatly increased. This is especially so for women, who are more than twice as likely to suffer from the disease. Weight-bearing exercise is one way to counter this.

When the bone is placed under stress, as in resistance training, there is a slight bend. This causes the builders in your bones (osteoblasts) to go to that area and release protein, which over time mineralizes to form new bone. The bone is larger and denser, so any force applied—and that includes hitting the sidewalk—is now spread over a larger area.

The increase in bone density is directly related to the area that you work. So for a stronger spine you need to apply a force to your back. X-rays show that the bones in a tennis player's favored arm are larger than those in the non-playing arm. Working all areas of the body will maintain a strong, healthy bone mass.

Mind as well as matter

The physical benefits of exercise are obvious. Most people exercise simply to lose weight and tone up. But what about the psychological benefits exercise offers?.

When you exercise, you are taking control of an aspect of your life without reference to anyone else. You are finding the time in your busy schedule to do something for yourself, knowing that it is going to make a difference. Exercise helps to relieve stress, helps you to focus, you will sleep better and you will feel generally much better about yourself. When you look in the mirror you will find a more positive you looking back. This might seem a little selfish, but the benefits of a more confident you will filter out to your loved ones, friends, and colleagues as well.

Regardless of whether you have lost weight, lifted more than last week, or just beaten the world bench pressing record, the simple fact that you are doing it *for you* is enough to start to change your self-image and spur you on to greater things.

Where can you train?

Anywhere. It all depends on how self-conscious or confident you are. You can exercise in specific environments such as gyms and aerobic classes. But with these come additional cost and occasional inconvenience.

Many people would like to exercise at home and with this book, you can. All you need is minimal equipment, some of which won't even cost you anything, a little space, and a willingness to try. You are familiar with your surroundings, you can have your own music playing, and you don't have to fight your way through a sweaty crowd for a place in the showers!

Who can train?

Just about everyone will benefit from resistance training. It is not only for those in pursuit of the body beautiful. Most lifestyles are not particularly active. We no longer have to hunt for our food, manual work is done by fewer and fewer, and our bodies have become lazy as a result. A weak and overweight body leads to health problems, as well

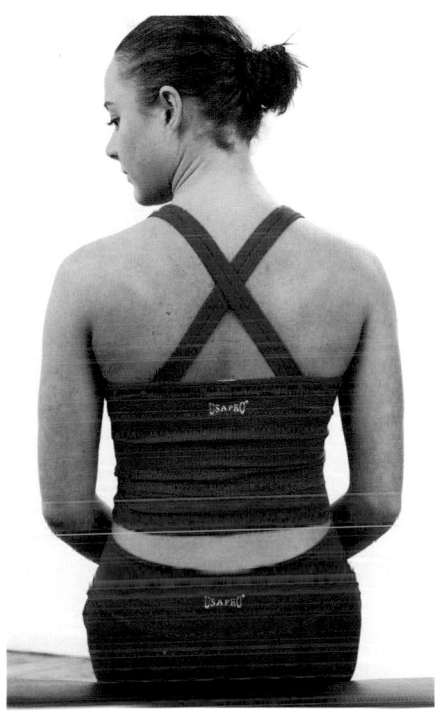

as giving people a negative image of themselves. So anything we do to counteract this is going to be beneficial. Resistance training is one of the best ways to fight back against the weakening effects of modern living. Regardless of sex, size, abilities, or disabilities, there is something to be gained for everyone.

But remember: if you have not exercised before, or have not done so for some time and are just starting out on a new regime, check with a health professional first. They will be able to give you a good idea of the level of intensity that you should be starting with. Once you have the all-clear, dive in and good luck.

Equipment

If you have ever walked in to a modern gym you will no doubt have been amazed at how much equipment people seem to need to keep fit and healthy. Millions of dollars are spent on gym equipment and as in all markets, products come and go. Last year's state-of-the-art treadmill is this year's bargain basement cast-off. The latest sensational abdominal exercise machine is quickly put aside to make way for something that looks equally odd. So how are you going to keep fit, tone up, and stay healthy without a budget of several thousand dollars? Use your imagination.

Look around your home and, unless you are exceptionally minimalist, it will be filled with all sorts of objects of varying sizes and weights. Some will be more useful than others. Tables, while heavy, are a little unwieldy if used as weights.

As well as those objects around the house there is equipment that you can buy that will not cost the earth, but will provide a lot more variety in your exercise routine. Here are the five best "home helps" and the five most recommended purchases.

In the home

Plastic drinks bottles The bottles themselves are very light but fill them up and they get heavy enough. And you can vary the weight through very small increments. There are of course many different sizes and shapes, some more convenient to handle than others. If you want a heavy weight go for the big ones with the carrying handle.

Chair or bench Thes provide the perfect base for working the backs of your arms when doing Dips and any seated weight work—so long they are sturdy and not of the type that folds up for storage.

Food cans Very similar to the plastic bottles except you cannot vary the contents and, therefore, the weight. Do not use glass jars for obvious reasons.

Plastic grocery bags Fill the bag with cans and you can now hold a variety of weights. In fact you could fill them up with pretty much anything. They may not be suitable for all the exercises, but they can certainly be of use.

Stairs Stair climbing is a very good form of exercise, working your thighs and your butt. Using the stairs will elevate your heart rate and body temperature in preparation for exercise.

Equipment best buys

Dumbbells Probably the single most useful piece of training kit that you can buy. These alone will make the exercise workouts more varied and make it easier to track your progress. Use the bottles of water if that is your only choice, but there is a measure of guesswork involved when it comes to how much they actually weigh.

The most common home dumbbells are fixed vinyl or neoprene. These are non-variable weight dumbbells that you usually buy in a set where the weight goes from 1 lb. to 10 lb., or 1 kg to 5 kg, in small increments. Heavier weights are available. The other types are plate-loaded dumbbells. Separate weight plates are put onto a metal bar to make a dumbbell that weighs however much you like. The plates themselves are either vinyl or metal, sometimes encased in rubber. The metal plates are smaller because the material they are made from is heavier. The down side is that it can be time-consuming to alter the weight between exercises.

This is where switchable-weight dumbbells come in. These are relatively new to the market. You simply move a lever or a pin and the weight changes without the need to remove or add plates for yourself. They sit in a specially designed base that holds the weights that are not being used. If you want more weight, simply return the dumbbell to the base, flick a switch, and it locks the additional weight in place. The advantage is that they are very easy to use and take up very little room when not in use. The down side is that they are a lot more expensive than the traditional style.

Exercise resistance bands or tubes

These are basically an industrial-strength elastic or latex band. The resistance is applied through stretching the band. They come in a range of styles and various tensions. The tension of the band is usually color-coded. A pink or yellow band will be easier than a red or a black band; but this may vary from manufacturer to manufacturer. The exercise tubes differ from the bands in that they have a handle on each end. Apart from this the principle is exactly the same.

Most dumbbell exercises can be recreated using the bands, as well as some that you cannot do with dumbbells. The bands are anchored at a point, be that your foot or a piece of (heavy) furniture, and pulled or pushed through a range of movement.

They are durable, but be careful after prolonged use. If the band or tube starts to split, it is time to throw it away and get a new one. It is not good when they snap in mid Lateral Raise! Taller people may find that they are limited by the length of the bands; because the bands will have to stretch more through

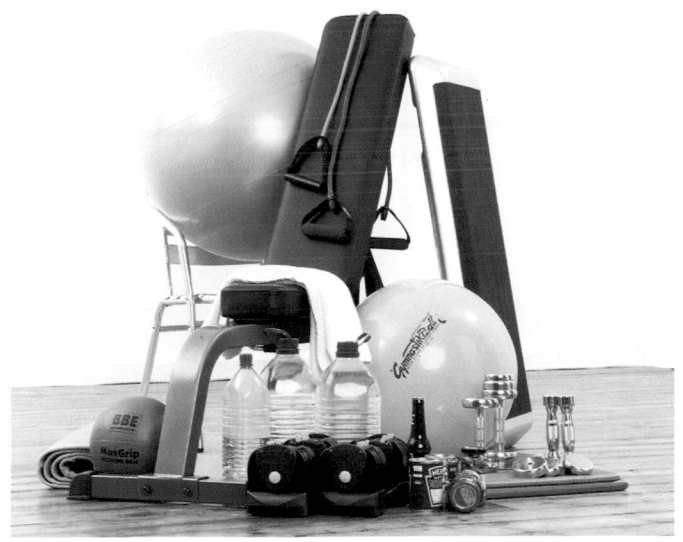

a range of movement the taller you are and the longer your limbs, there will be more resistance. This can be a limiting factor. One great plus point is that bands take up practically no storage space and are easily portable for travel.

Stability, or Swiss Balls Combine one of these with a pair of dumbbells and your potential for variety is almost infinite. In terms of resistance training the ball can play many roles. It can take the place of a bench or seat for horizontal and sitting positions. The ball on its own can be used as a pivot point for some exercises involving your body weight. Because it is a ball you are forced to stabilize your body. This means more muscle recruitment, better posture, and potentially more calories used during the workout. By its very nature, the ball can give softer, more pliable support than a bench, which can be useful for some exercises.

The stability balls come in many different sizes, so there will be one that suits you. The only problem with Swiss balls is storage. They can, though, be inflated and deflated in minutes using a good pump.

Training Bench A bench provides you with a station on which to exercise. It means that you are not on the floor and gives you the stability that a household chair or bench may not. It positions you at a height that will suit almost all exercises during the workout.

For the majority of exercises a simple, flat bench is adequate. You can, however, buy benches with various features, the most common one being an incline. This allows you to position

the bench at any angle between flat and straight up. This can be an advantage for some exercises but is by no means essential.

Like the stability ball, the down side is storage. You can buy benches that will fold up to a size approaching an ironing board, so if storage is an issue, ask about this feature before you buy.

Medicine Ball The medicine ball has moved on from the old days when it terrorized you or your dad in the school gym if wielded by an over-enthusiastic teacher. They now comes in various materials. You can still buy them in their traditional leather form, but you can now buy rubber balls. These are much smaller while still being heavy, making them much more versatile. Some medicine balls even have handles to make it easier to hold them.

The balls come in a variety of weights ranging from 2 lb. (1 kg) to over 20 lb. (10 kg). Buying a range of medicine balls can be expensive. To keep the cost down the best thing to do is buy a weight that is going to be suitable for the most exercises, compromising on a few. They are great for abdominal work and more sport-orientated drills.

The equipment that would help you to take full advantage of the exercises given here—and allow for more progression if desired—is a good set of dumbbells and a stability ball or bench. This combination will allow you to work every muscle in your body without the need to buy any other equipment ever again: except maybe heavier dumbbells after following the exercises and recommendations given.

Pre-and Post-workout

Before you begin to exercise it is very important to prepare the body for the higher intensity work that it will be asked to do. The warm-up is intended to have four beneficial effects:

1 To elevate the heart rate smoothly, without any sudden increases;
2 Gradually to increase core body temperature;
3 To increase muscle temperature and elasticity;
4 To mobilize and "lubricate" joints.

The stretching exercises pictured on pages 22 to 25 are strongly recommended not just as part of the warm-down but also as part of *any* exercise and fitness regime. The warm-down, among other benefits:

1 Increases the range of movement of the muscles and in so doing reduces the potential for later muscle soreness;
2 Like stretching at any time, increases flexibility and improves balance over time;
3 Reduces the level of adrenaline in the blood;
4 Helps you psychologically to prepare to return to the outside world! This should not be underestimated after a challenging workout.

Warm-up

Think of it this way: your workout does not start *with* a warm-up, it starts *at* the warm-up. That way you will not see it as a chore, or as a waste of time.

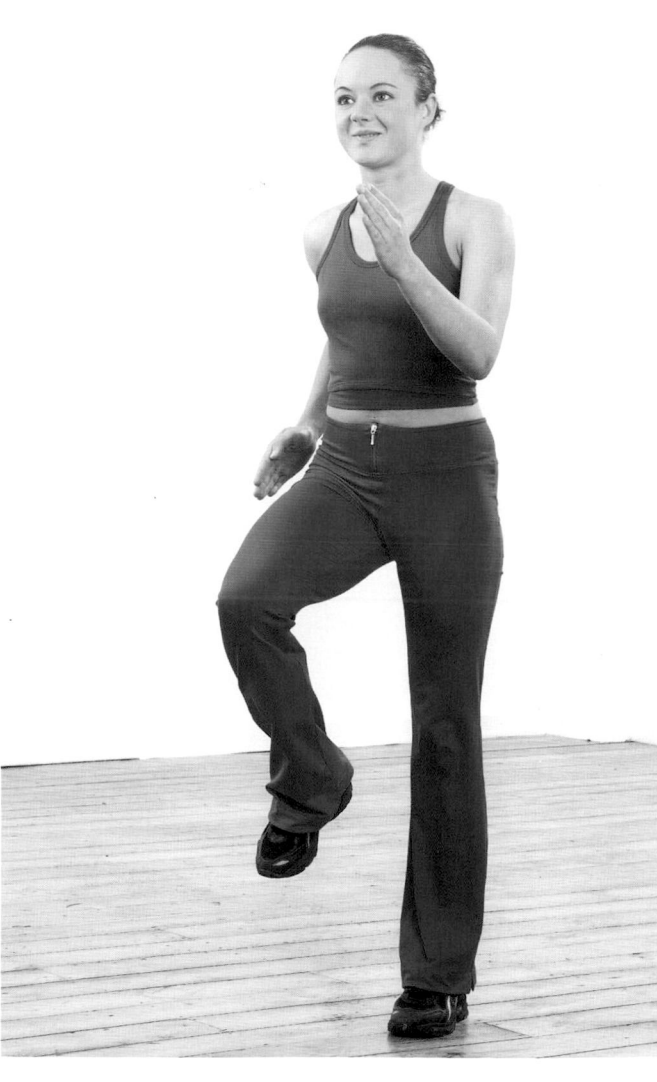

The first aim is to increase heart rate and core body temperature. As you move your body, your muscles contract and relax. Every time they contract there is a chemical reaction and more blood has to go to the muscle. As more blood is required in the muscle, your heart rate increases. As a result the temperature of the muscle gradually increases.

It is important that the emphasis is on "gradually." The minimum time for a warm-up should be around five minutes but ideally a little more. This will depend on the individual (are you generally a warm person?), the temperature of your training environment, clothing, etc. Starting too quickly, too soon, is one of the reasons many people do not continue with exercise. Remember that your heart is a muscle. And it is one muscle you really don't want to pull! Begin slowly, get the blood into the muscles, and start to feel warmer.

The initial few minutes of exercise can feel the most uncomfortable, as your body is working uneconomically. Start at a low intensity and give your body a chance. The activity will gradually feel much more comfortable. In the latter stages of the warm-up slowly increase the intensity to near the level at which the main workout will

1 The obvious start. Move the arms.

take place. If the main workout is going to be a continuation of the warm-up, then the approach is straightforward. For example, a running warm-up would go something like this:

1 Moderate pace walk (three minutes)
2 Brisk walk increasing stride length (two minutes)
3 Light jog (three minutes)
4 Fast jog increasing stride length (two minutes)
5 Light run (three minutes)
6 Running at workout pace (duration of workout)

It's very simple. Start slowly and build up. As the intensity increases at a gradual pace, your body is not as shocked as if going straight into a run. If you have ever had to run for a train, you will know exactly how uncomfortable it is, suddenly to go from rest to full throttle.

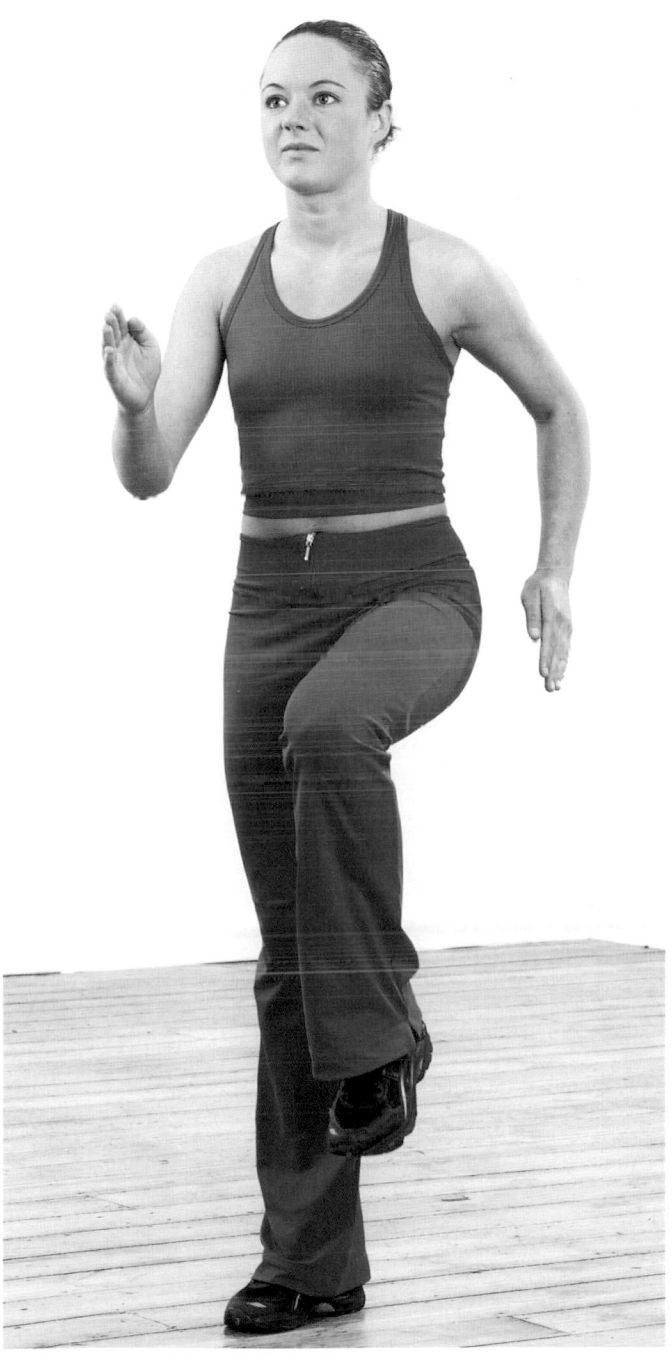

2 Gradually lift the knees higher.

Warm-up

After marching, the next logical body wake-up call is the Side Step, combined with arm curls for the biceps and triceps.

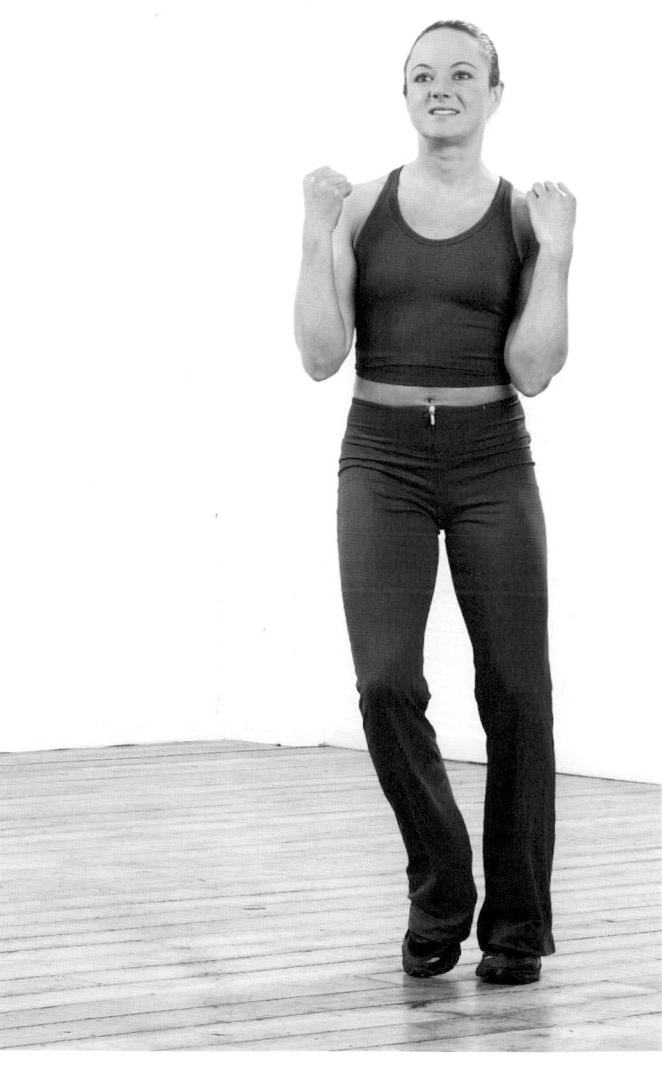

The second aim is to increase muscle temperature and elasticity. Muscles like to be warm. They work better that way. They contract faster and can release oxygen at a much quicker rate than when cold. These two factors alone are worth warming up for—but there is another good reason.

The muscles in your body are a little like Play-Doh. If they are cold they tend not to want to stretch too far before tearing. With Play-Doh this isn't such a bad thing as you can stick it back together and start again. This is not an option with your muscles, so tears and pulls are best avoided. Like the Play-Doh, once you have warmed the muscles up they become much more pliable and are content to go through the range of movement that the strength training exercises are about to put them through.

1 Side Step; start with hands up.

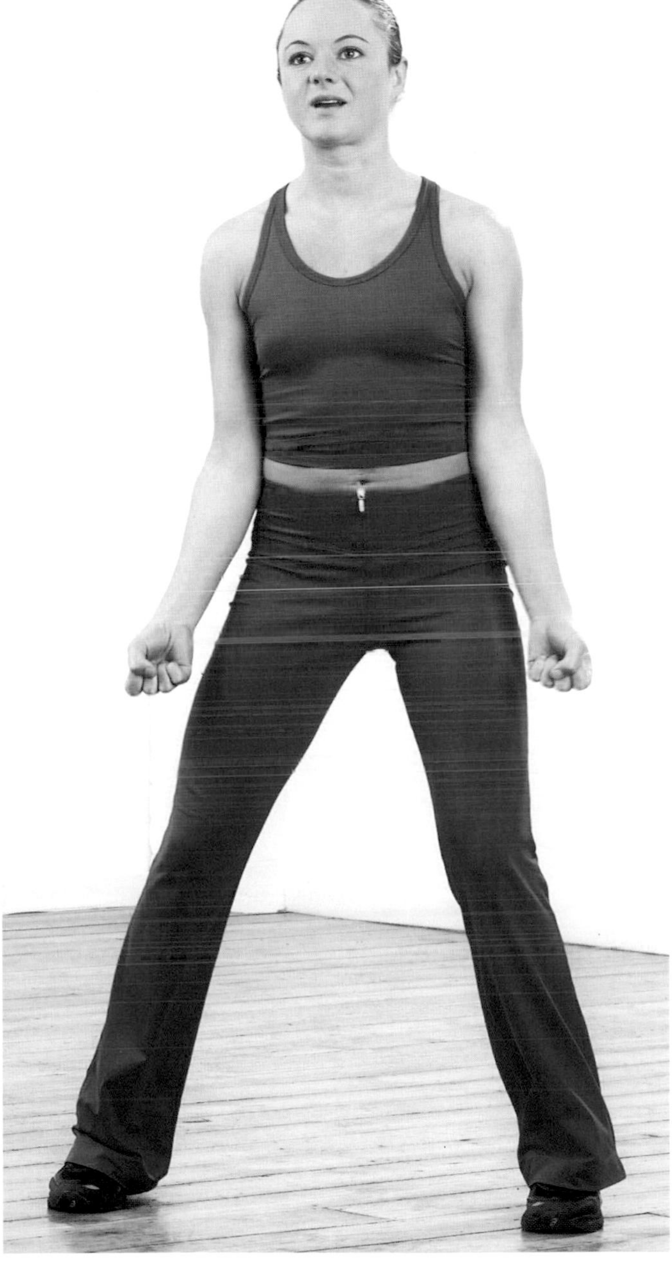

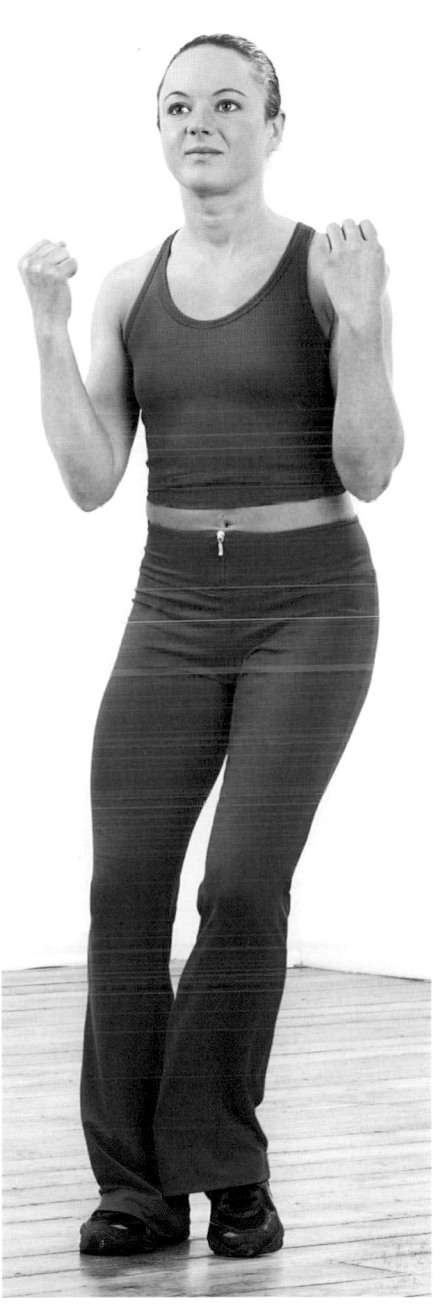

2 Step wider than shoulder-width.

3 Even your abs begin to get involved.

Warm-up

Mobilizing the joints is the third aim of the warm-up. While side stretching and nudging the upper back awake, Half Jacks also mobilize the knee joints and loosen the shoulders.

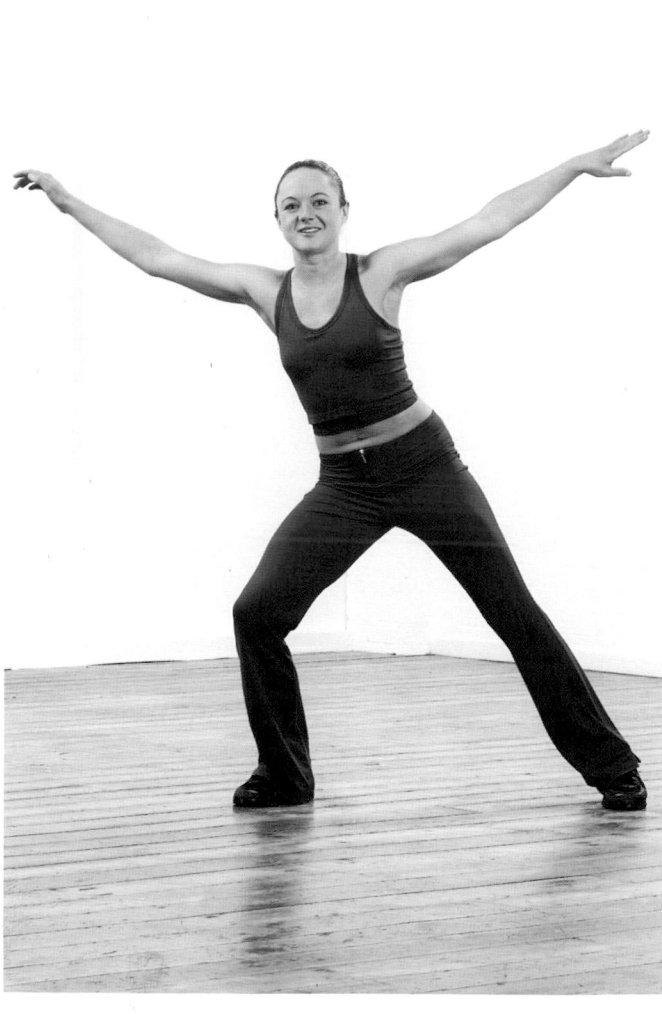

When you get up in the morning, or after you have been sitting for too long, your joints may feel stiff. One reason for this is that your muscles have been in a single position for some time and may be a little tight. Another reason is that your joints haven't moved either and need a bit of natural oil to help them on their way.

Movement of a joint produces synovial fluid. This is the body's answer to engine oil and helps to reduce friction within the joint, resulting in it feeling much easier to move. Cartilage that covers the end of the bones absorbs some of this fluid, causing it to expand and become thicker, making it better at shock absorbance.

It is important that the joint is taken through the same movement that will be done at a higher intensity. This means that there are no surprises once the weight is increased and a greater load is applied to the joint. Before lifting weights, go through the range of movement several times to make sure that the muscles and joints are activated. There is also less chance of injury this way, rather than going straight in and lifting the weight. This will also prepare you psychologically for the exercise, as you will be going through exactly the same range of movement as in the main workout.

1 Half Jack; next stage of the Side Step.

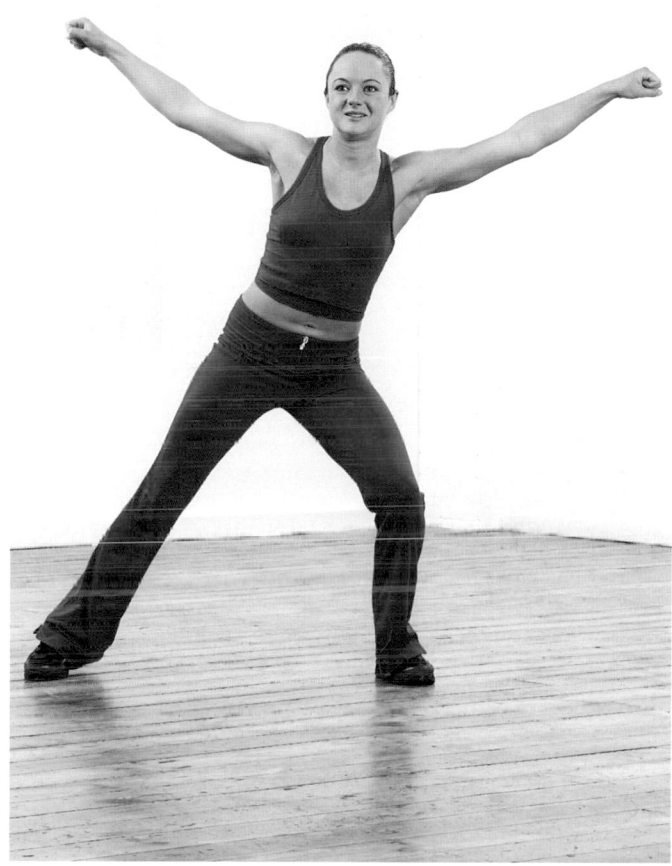

3 Hands to shoulder height or just above.

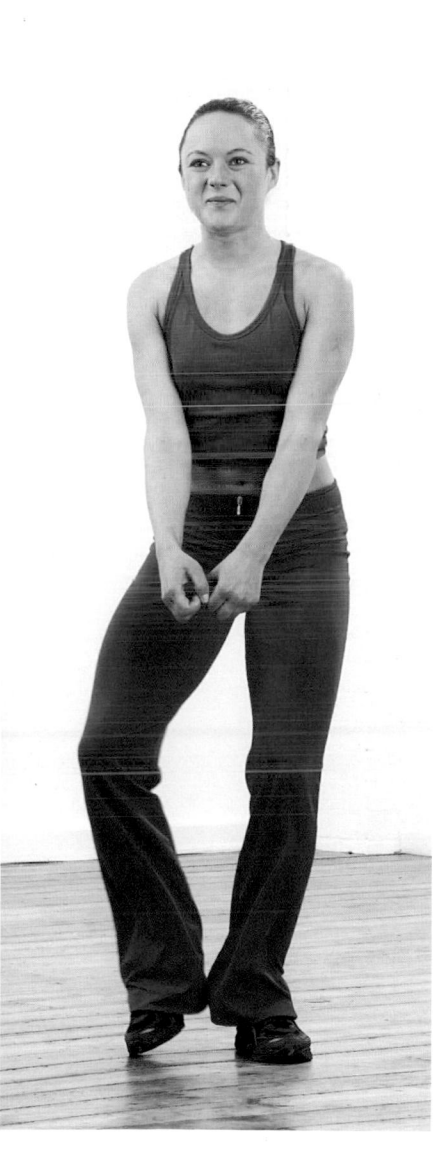

2 Relaxed hands to the center.

Warm-up

The warm-up involves the use of all the main joints and muscles. It is not just about avoiding injury: as important is avoiding the shock of a "cold start" that might put you off training.

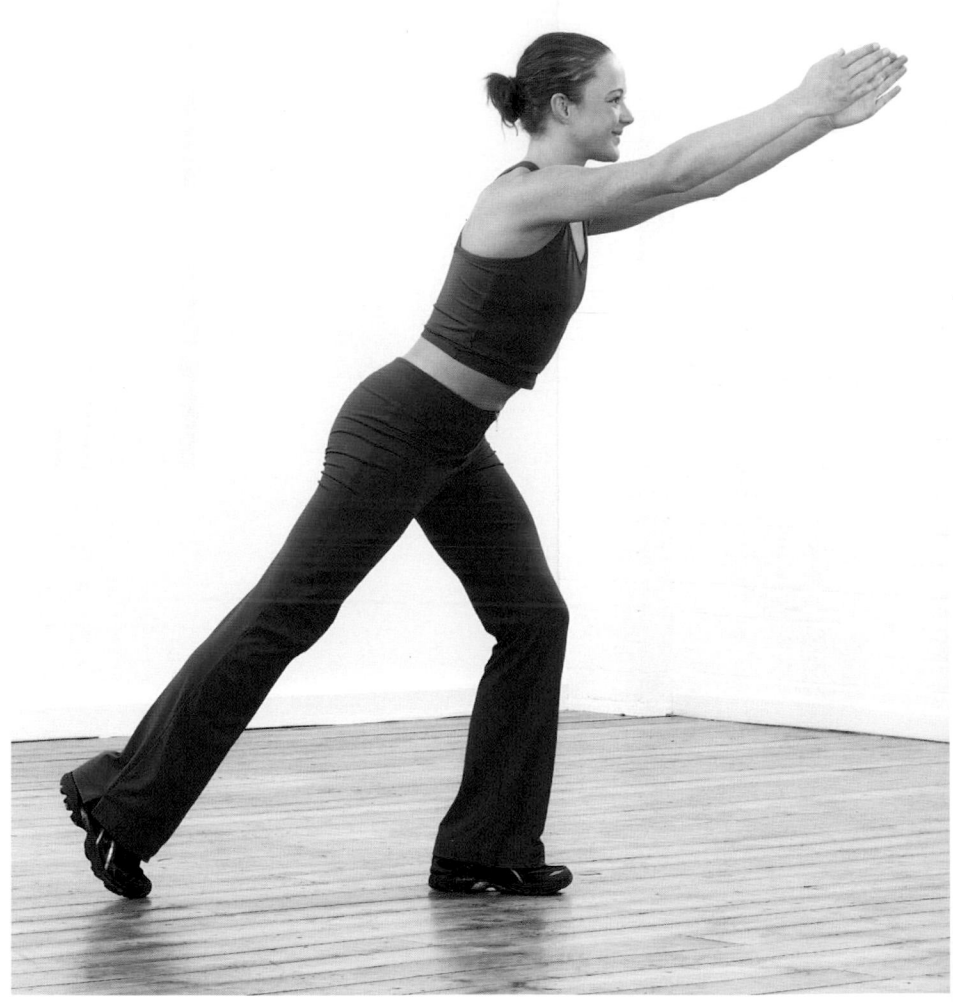

1 Rear Lunge (+ arm raise); an exaggerated step back, landing on the ball of the foot

2 The knees are slightly bent.

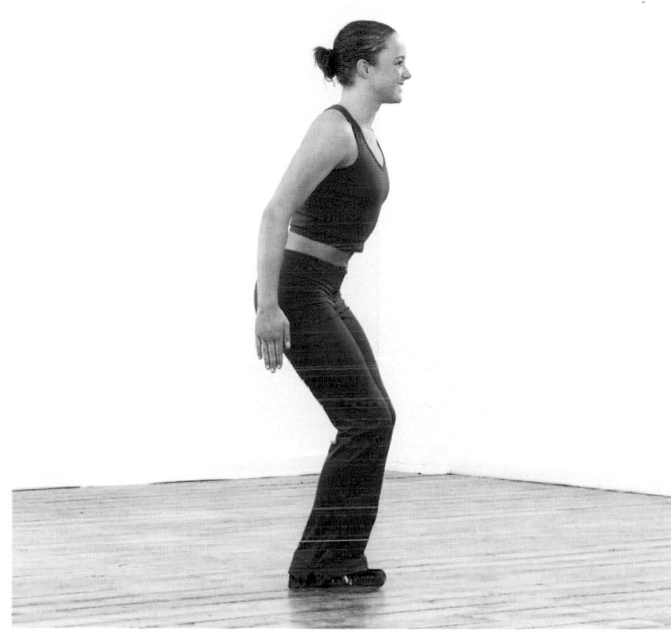

The following exercises help to prepare the body for the weight training routines. It is good to have music playing while you exercise if you can. Select something that motivates you. Something a little bouncy with a strong beat can help, as this will make it easier to work the steps to.

1 Marching on the Spot x 16
2 Side Step (right leg leading) x 8
3 Side Step (left leg leading) x 8
4 Marching on the spot, knees lifting higher x 16
5 Side Step, stepping wider (right leg leading) x 8 + Ankle Rotations (right foot) x 4
6 Side Step (left leg leading) x 8 + Ankle Rotations (left foot) x 4
7 Marching on Spot (knees lifting higher) x 16
8 Half Jacks (arms to shoulder height) x 8.
9 Rear Lunge (alternating) + Front Arms Raise x 8

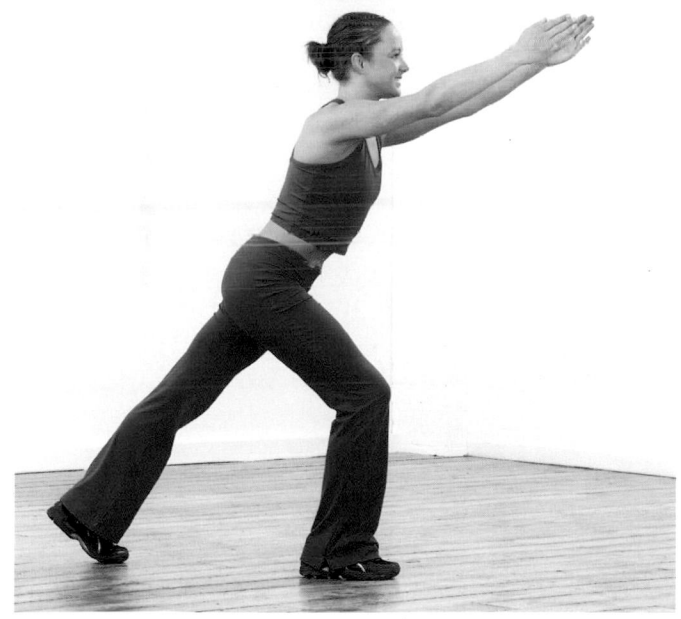

3 The front knee is not over the toes.

Warm-down

Allow enough time for a warm-down. If you are new to strength exercises, warm-down from the very first workout and it will soon become second nature.

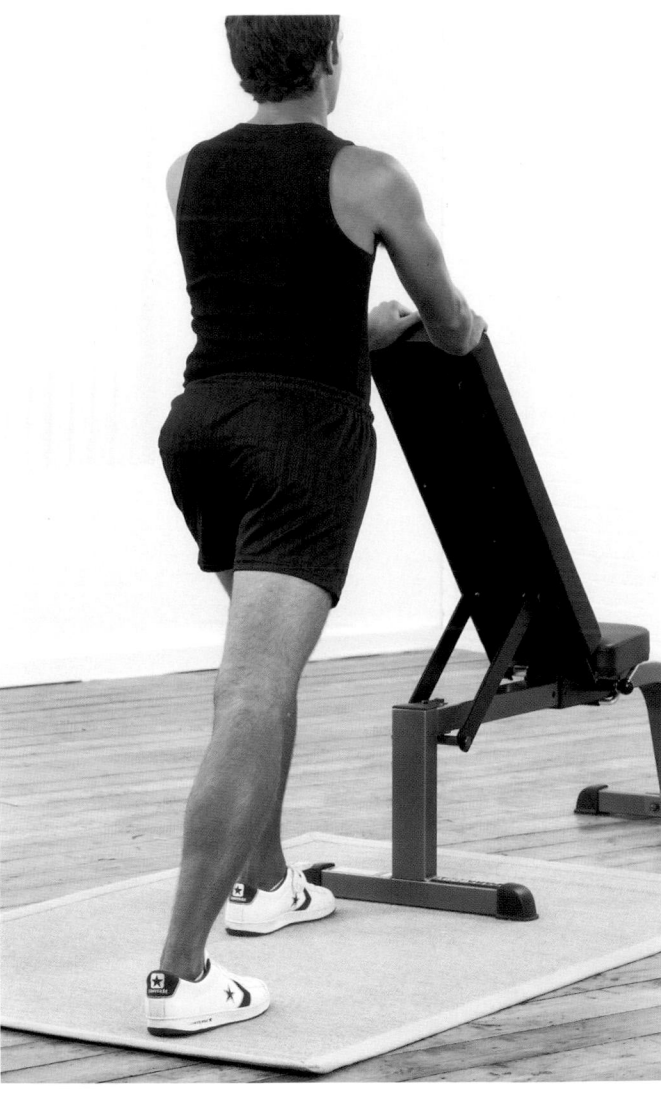

It is tempting to get to the end of your workout and make a dash for the shower before the rest of your life suddenly comes hurtling back into your day. Wait. Have you given your body a chance to come back to normality?

Just like the warm-up, you need to gradually bring your body back down to a near pre-exercise state. So if you have been really going for it in your workout, gently come back down. Go through the warm-up workout again, but instead of gradually increasing intensity, decrease it. You should still feel warm as you will need to retain your elevated core temperature to stretch, but you should not be out of breath or perspiring.

By the nature of resistance training the workouts can leave you with a lot of tension and tightness in the muscles that have been working. It is thought by some that post-workout stretches may help to minimize delayed onset muscle soreness (DOMS). The warm-down aids the dissipation of waste products from the muscles, including lactic acid, and provides time for a reduction in the level of adrenaline in the blood.

Back/lower leg stretch. Heel flat, a sma step back from a support.

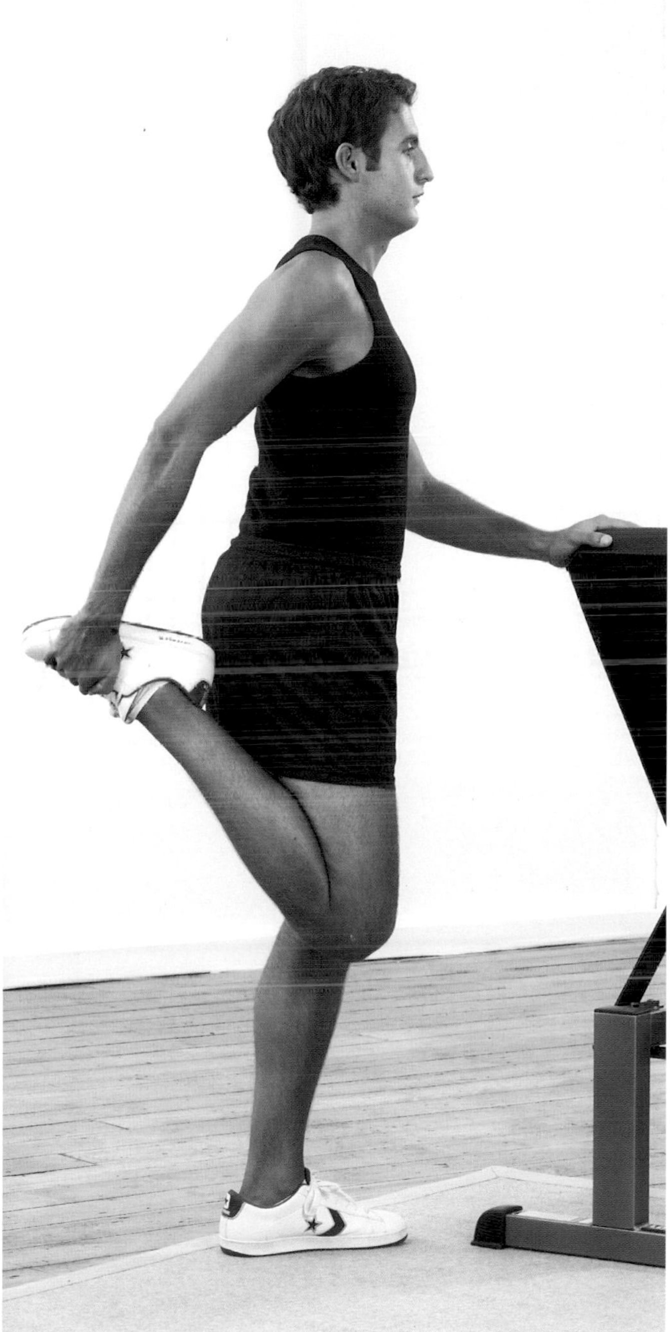

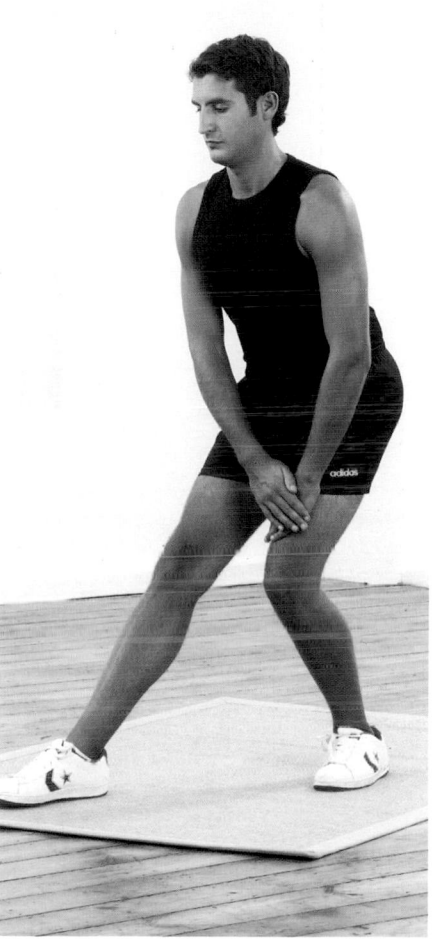

Above: Back of thigh.

Left: Front of thigh.

Warm-down

These stretches lengthen all the main muscle groups. The warm-down reduces the risk of dizziness or fainting caused by the pooling of blood in the extremities.

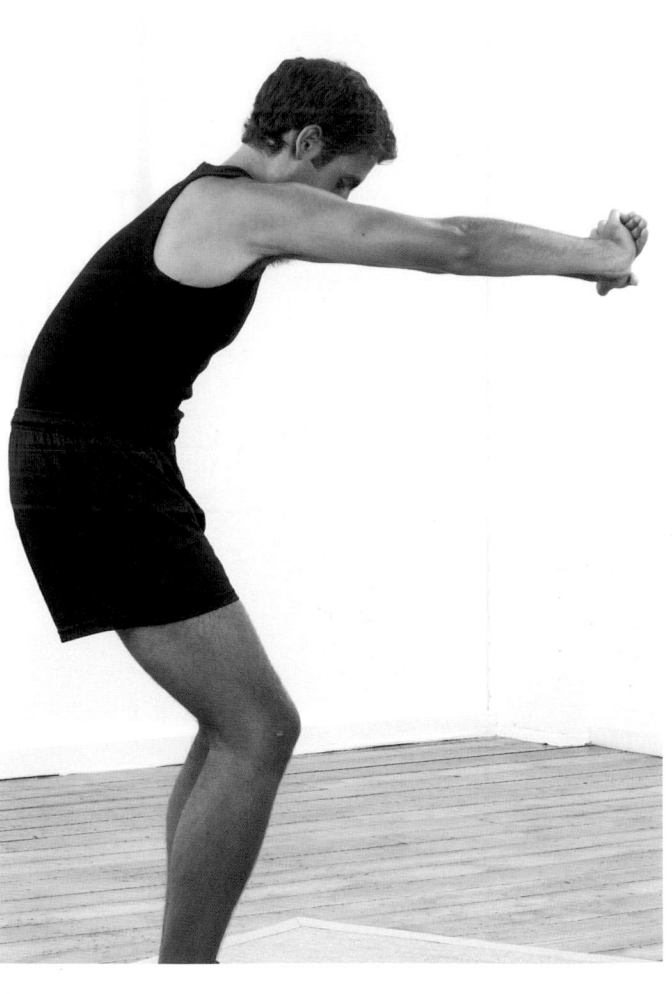

At the very end of your workout, go through the following basic stretches. Hold each one for 10–20 seconds and repeat two or three times. When you stretch you should feel the muscle lengthen. Hold it at the point of mild discomfort. If you are gritting your teeth and your eyes begin to water, you may be taking the stretch a little too far! Static stretches are appropriate for the warm-down as they relax the muscles and help to increase their range of movement.

1   Back of lower leg
     (Gastrocnemius)
2   Front of thigh (Quadriceps)
3   Back of thigh (Hamstring)
4   Upper back (Trapezius, Erector Spinae)
5   Chest and front of shoulder (Pectoral, Anterior Deltoid)
6   Sides and upper back (Latissimus Dorsi)
7   Back of arm (Triceps)

Upper back. Alternate hand positions.

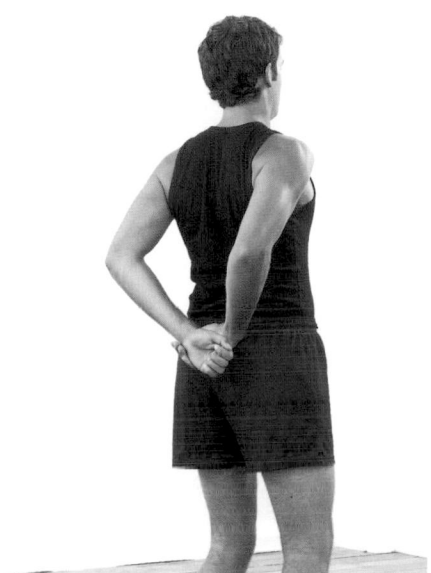

Chest and front of shoulder.

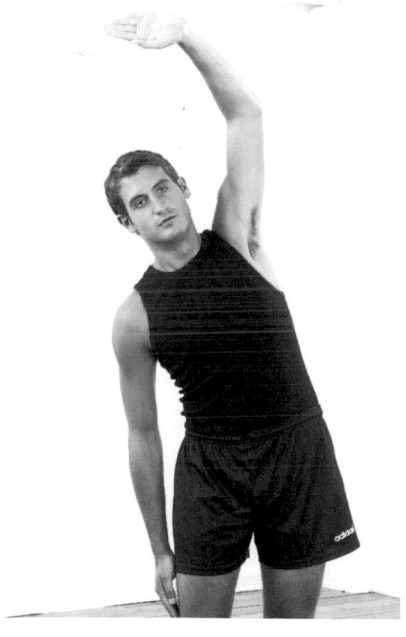

Sides and upper back.

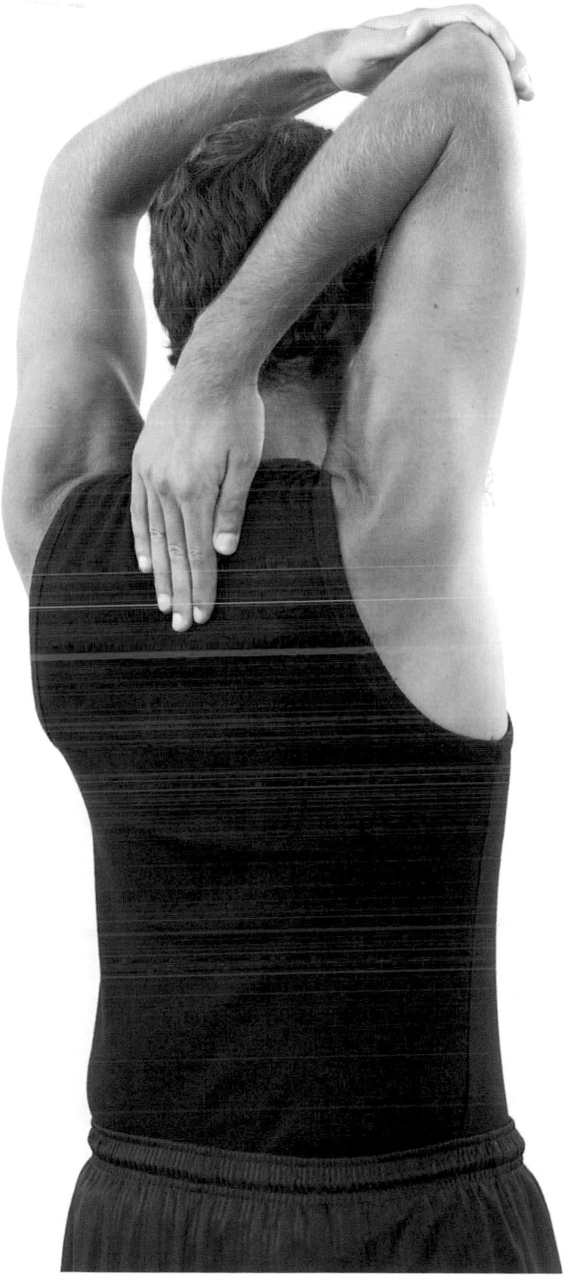

Back of arm. Push down gently and hold.

Training Principles

Monitor your progress. Keep a workout log with how many repetitions and what weight you lifted. Keep an eye on how your clothes are fitting!

There are certain elements that should stay constant throughout your training and some things that you should vary. Things that you vary will affect the intensity of the workout, making it easier or harder. Things to try to keep constant are the following:

Range of Movement You will develop strength only in the range of movement that you lift through. This means that you need to go all the way up and all the way down. This does make the exercise harder as it is more difficult to lift a weight from the lowest point, but it does mean that you will yield greater gains in the long run. Do not sacrifice your range of movement in an attempt to lift more weight. Move through a range of movement that you feel comfortable with. If it feels wrong or there is pain or discomfort that is not related to the exercise, often in a joint, then adjust. There is no unchallenged textbook way. Everyone is built that little bit differently, so what feels right for one person may not feel right for the next.

Repetition Speed How fast you lift affects how hard your muscle will work. The faster you go the more momentum is generated. The more momentum is generated, then the less work your muscles have to do. The less work your muscles do, the less gains you make. Simple. But how fast should you lift? There is still some debate about this; but

for the majority of the population and for the recreational exerciser (those of us who are not athletes) it is recommended that the lifting (concentric) phase of the movement should last approximately two seconds and the lowering (eccentric) phase should last from three to four seconds. Your muscles can actually lower more weight than they can lift so if in doubt remember, "lower = slower." As your muscles become tired, the temptation is to increase your speed, especially in the lowering phase. When lowering, try to think of it as a smooth release of pressure, rather then a sudden release. A little like applying the brakes in the car: but not an emergency stop!

Posture Most injuries in the gym are posture-related. Poor posture means a weakened position and when you are lifting a weight, or acting against a resistance, this is not a good combination. Within many of today's working environments (such as desk-based computing) and with general lifestyle demands (commuting, driving, etc.) most people suffer from poor posture because they are sitting down much of the time. This can lead to a postural change where the upper portion (thoracic) part of the spine curves excessively, the head projects forward, and the shoulders droop forward. Resistance training can help reduce this, as can a good mobility and flexibility program. When exercising,

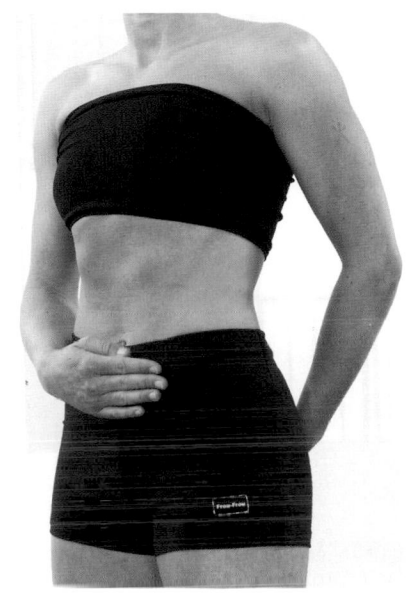

always make the following posture checks before you start to lift.

- Feet slightly wider than width between the hips.
- Knees soft when standing.
- Abdominal muscles braced, not pushed out.
- Chest lifted.
- Shoulders set back.
- Eyes forward, chin lifted.
- Think of it as standing tall.

Improving your posture instantly makes you look taller and slimmer. Develop a routine where you are reminding yourself of this on a regular basis. At first it has to be a conscious effort, but eventually over time having good posture is something you won't even think about, it will just happen.

The variables

These are the elements in your workouts that can be altered to change how hard the workout is. The variable you use is up to you, but try one at a time, as they can make a big difference:

Weight This initially will be your variable. As you become stronger, you are able to lift more weight and work using a greater resistance. When you do decide that you are going to increase the resistance, remember to make small adjustments. Think of it as a staircase to climb. You could get to the top in maybe a few big jumps but if you slipped the fall would hurt. Take it a step at a time and while it may take a little longer, you still reach the same point in one piece. But remember that this is not your only form of progression. It is easy to forget there are others.

Multiple Sets This is another area where debate still rages. Current research shows that for most recreational exercise one set of an exercise to momentary muscular fatigue yields nigh on the same gains as that of multiple sets. So from a time point of view, single-set training will give you optimum results. While this is true for strength gains, doing more sets will use more calories as a whole, though it will mean that you spend longer exercising. This calorie-burning may be an element to consider in the future, but in the beginning use the single set principle.

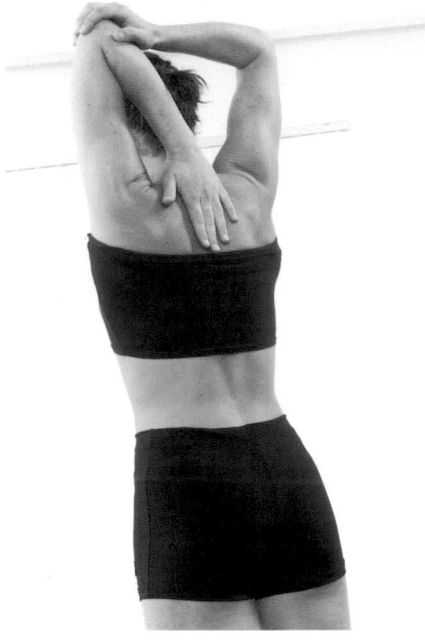

Dumbbell Row works the back and biceps. This allows one set of muscles to work while the other is recovering.

Tri-Sets Not to be confused with the muscle on the back of your arms. The thinking behind the Tri-Set is similar to that for Supersets. Rather than working opposing muscles you do three (hence "tri-set") exercises for the same muscle group, working it through three different types of movement. For example, for your legs you might do a Squat, a Lunge, and a Calf Raise. Your back would be Towel Pulldowns, Dumbbell Row, and a Pullover; again, all with as little rest in between as possible.

Rest Time Varying your rest time has a great effect on the intensity of the exercise. Resting in between exercises allows you to recover and prepare for the next exercise. But if you had already set the next exercise, or several exercises, you could reduce your rest time and work faster between them, thus making the workout as a whole much harder. There are several recognized forms of resistance training that use this principle.

Order of Exercise This is an often forgotten method of making things harder. If you use different muscles on each exercise then each muscle gets a rest before it has to work again. If you work the same muscle for two exercises it is still going to be slightly fatigued, so you have to work harder to complete the set. If your routine goes something like chest, back, legs, chest, back, shoulders, then try switching it to chest, chest, legs, shoulders, back, back, to make the routine harder. Your body needs change to adapt. Without change your body has no reason to, and therefore will not, adapt. These adaptations are directly affected by your use of the variables.

Supersets A traditional superset is comprised of two exercises for opposing muscles with no rest between them. This, in theory, means that by doing the first exercise you will have mobilized and warmed up the joints and muscles for the next exercise. An example of a superset would be a Press Up followed by a Dumbbell Row. The Press Up works the chest and triceps while the

The Exercises

Look back at the running warm-up example on page 15 and consider the different durations of the activities—resistance training and running. To complete a good run you may be looking at anything up to an hour and maybe more. When lifting a weight, a single set will probably take you a minute. Therefore, selecting the correct weight is very important. Too light and you will not achieve the desired effect; too much and you will burn out too quickly, like running for that train. So when lifting the weight it should feel something like this:

1 Reps 1–4: comfortable.
2 Reps 5–6: weight should start to feel a little heavy.
3 Reps 7–8: effort now required to keep the weight moving.
4 Reps 9–10: a lot of effort required to lift the weight.
5 Reps 11–12: just able to lift with good technique; but more repetitions and the technique would suffer.

As in the running warm-up, you are looking for small increments of intensity, but in this case over a matter of seconds rather than minutes, so be aware of this when choosing your working weight. If in doubt, start lighter, as this will reduce your chance of injury.

Chest–Beginners

half press up

Area Worked: Chest, front of shoulders, and back of arms.
Name of Muscles: Pectoralis, Anterior Deltoid, and Triceps.

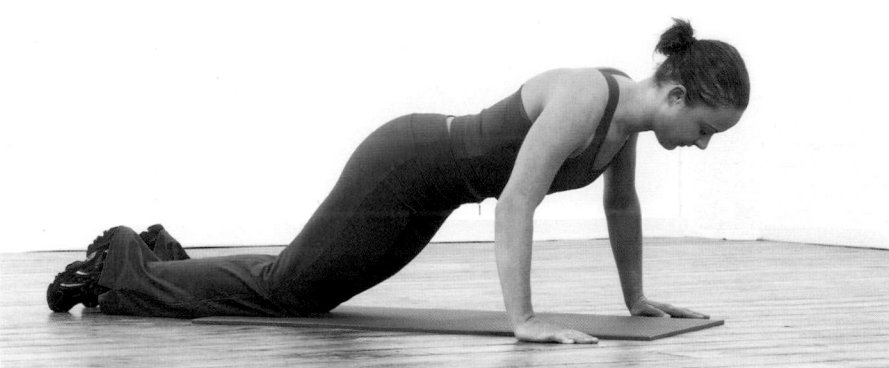

1 Kneel on the floor on all fours, placing your hands slightly wider than your shoulders.

2 Shuffle your knees back until your back is flat and horizontal.

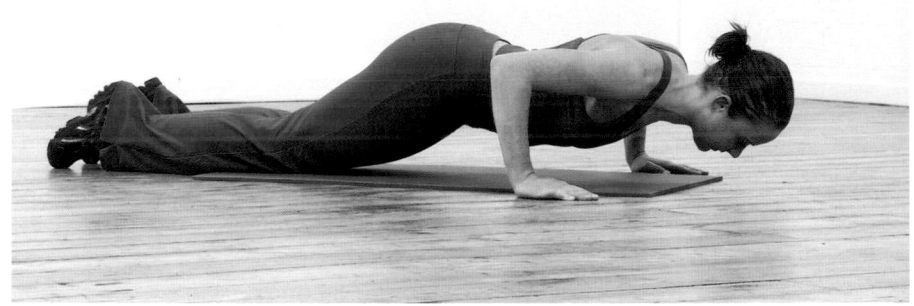

Hints & Tips

• Keep your whole body braced with your weight over your arms. It is tempting to let your weight shift back to make the exercise easier. Keep your hands in line with your chest.

• Keep thinking, "Tight abs, tight abs..."

Technique

- Never lock out your elbows. Keep the joint soft at all times.

- When moving your knees back, make sure you only move your knees, not your whole body. Your hands should be level with your chest throughout the exercise.

- Your abdominal muscles are working all the time throughout this exercise, so keep them braced tight. Don't push them out—pull them in!

- For the first few repetitions keep the range of movement small and gradually increase it. Aim to get your chest to within a couple of inches from the floor before pushing back up.

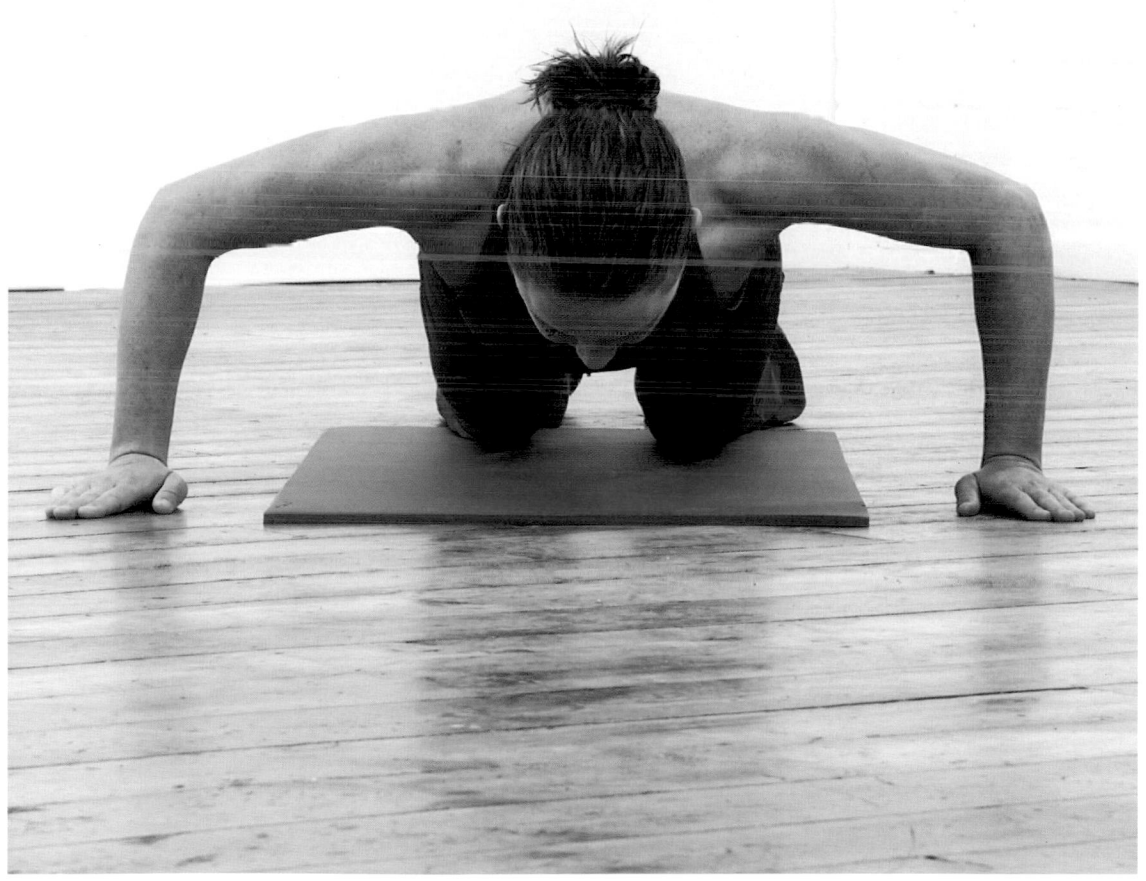

3 By bending your elbows lower your chest toward the floor, then by pushing your hands against the floor straighten your arms again.

Chest–Beginners

bench press

Area Worked: Chest, front of shoulders, and back of arms.
Name of Muscles: Pectoralis, Anterior Deltoid, and Triceps.

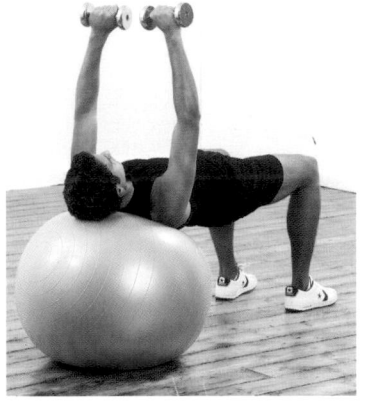 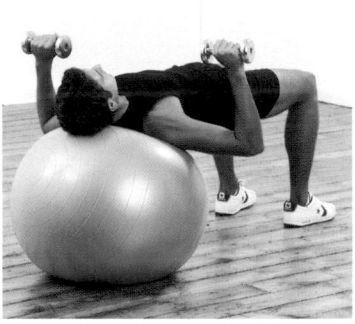 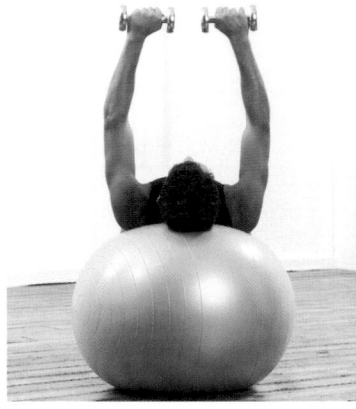

1 Lie with your feet flat and your legs slightly wider than your hips. Hold the weights over your chest with your palms forward.

2 Bending the elbows, lower the weights down toward your chest.

3 Push the dumbbells up, straightening the arms, until you are back in the start position.

Hints & Tips

• The weights should feel balanced. If you feel that your arms are being pulled back over your head move them further down your body; the opposite if they are being pulled forward.

• Your forearms should always be vertical throughout the movement. Do not let your hands drift inward or outward, as this puts extra strain on muscles other than the ones that you are trying to work.

Technique

- Keep the body braced and tensed all the time. This gives you a stable base from which to do the exercise.

- The weights over the chest should have a small gap between them at the start and finish of each repetition.

- Think of the movement as a triangle with slightly curved sides. The top of the movement is the point of the triangle, and the bottom of the movement is the base of the triangle; your weights are moving between these two points in a smooth arc.

- Be careful when straightening the arms that you don't lock them out. Keep the elbows soft.

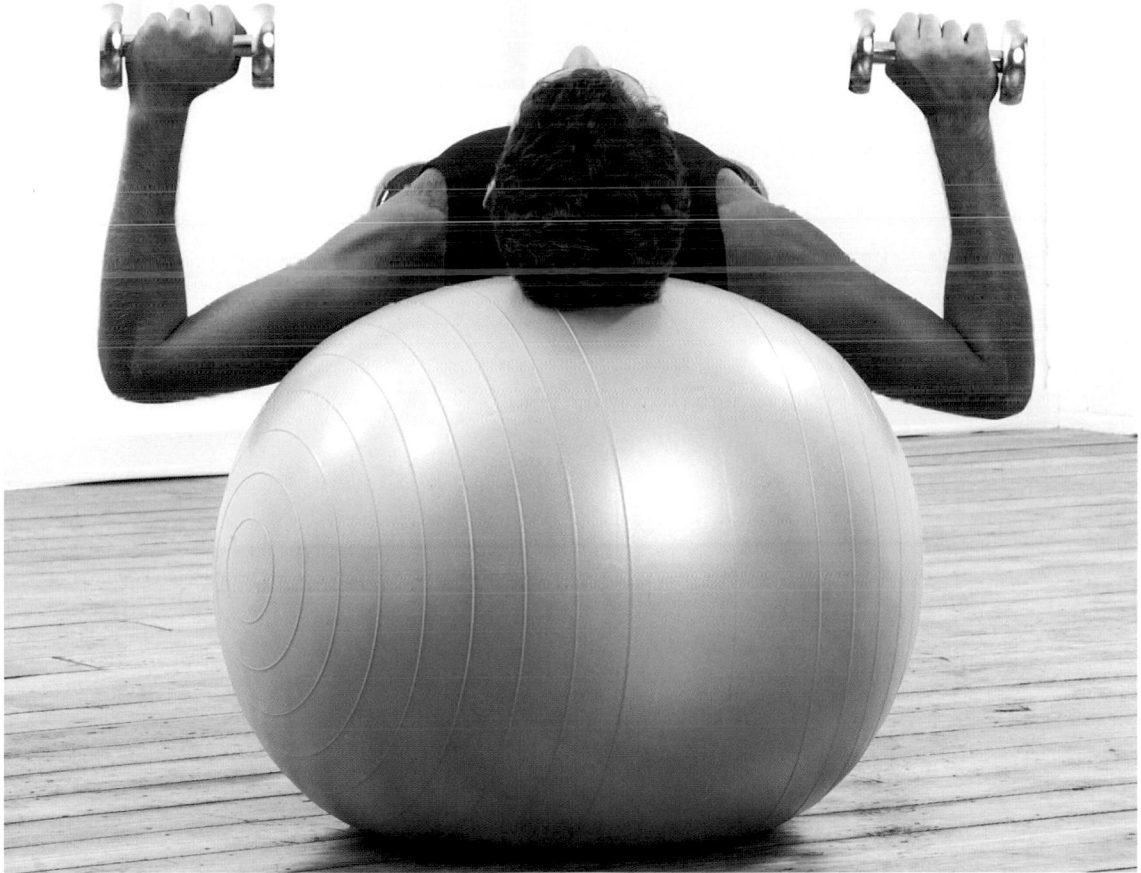

4 Keep your forearms vertical throughout, particularly at the bottom of the movement, as this ensures the hands do not move in or away from the body.

Chest—Beginners

pectoral fly

Area Worked: Chest.
Name of Muscle: Pectoralis.

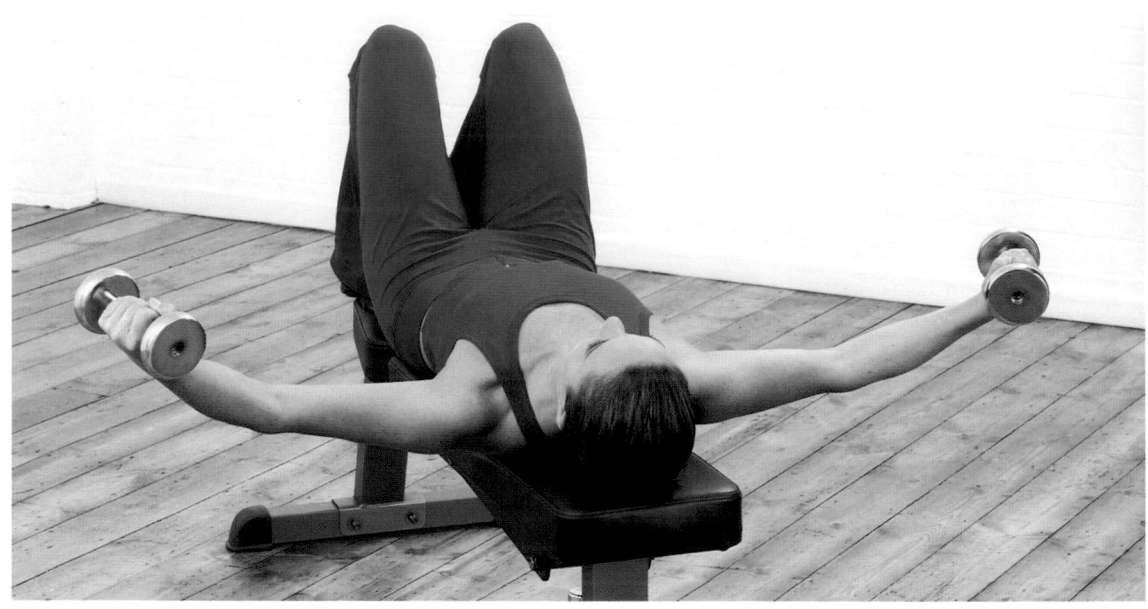

1 Lay on the floor/ball/bench with your feet flat and your legs slightly wider than your hips. Hold the weights over your chest with palms facing inward. Lower the arms out to the side in a smooth arc.

Hints & Tips

- Try to visualize your pectoral muscles squeezing together to bring the weights back in to the chest.

- Try to keep the grip as relaxed as you can, to keep focus on the chest—without dropping the weights!

Technique

- Keep the body braced and tensed all the time. This gives you a stable base from which to do the exercise.

- The weights over the chest should have a small gap between them at the start and finish of each repetition.

- When lowering the weights out to the side keep them in line with the chest and make sure that the slight bend in the elbow is maintained throughout the movement.

- Be careful how far you lower the weights initially. The weights should just be above being level with your chest when taken out to the sides, but this may vary according to your flexibility.

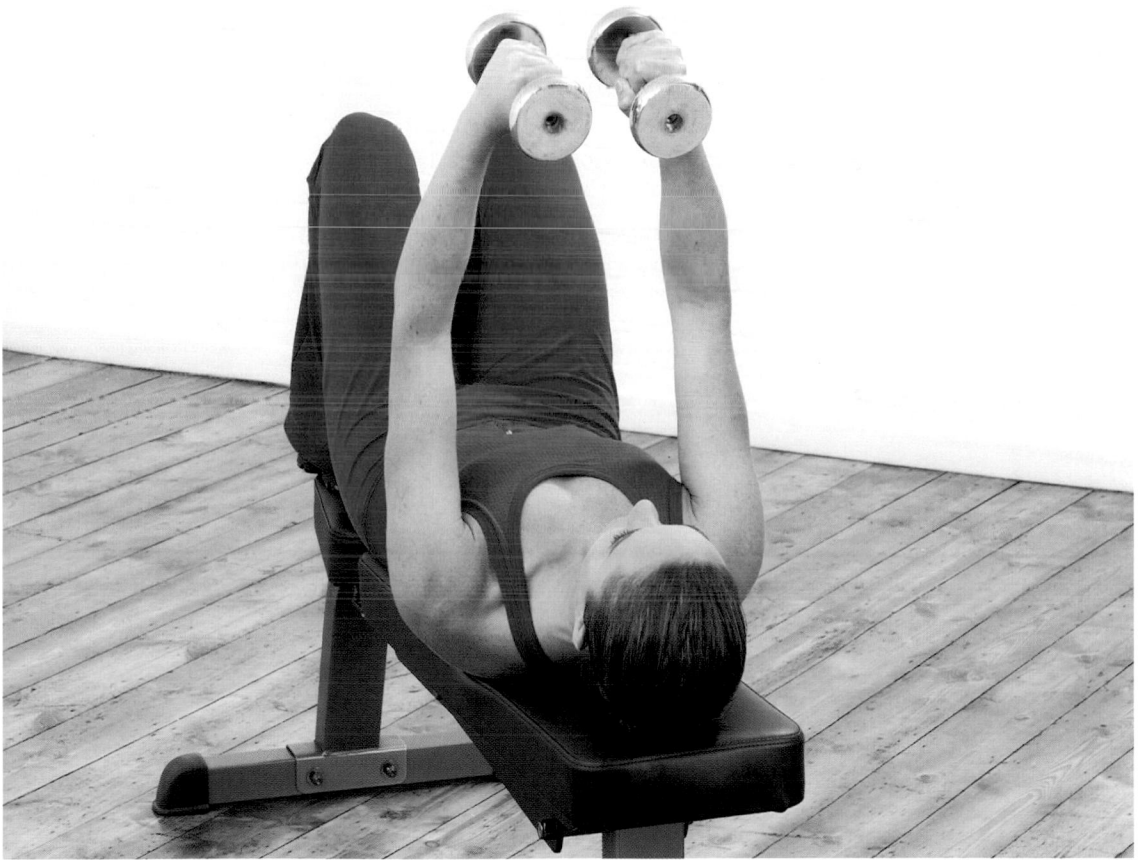

2 Place a slight bend in the elbows so that they are not locked. Return the weights back to the starting position.

Chest–Advanced

full/three-point press up

Area Worked: Chest, front of shoulders, and back of arms.
Name of Muscles: Pectoralis, Anterior Deltoid, and Triceps (Abdominal stabilizing).

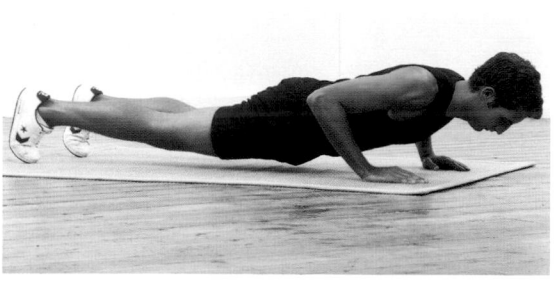

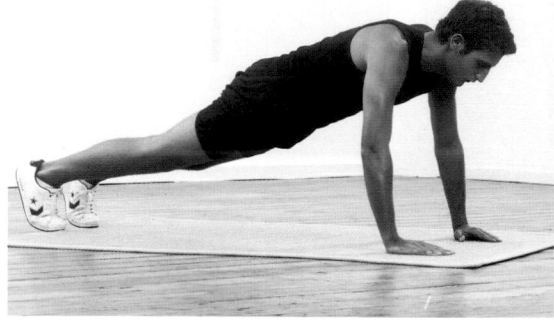

1   Lie face down on the floor, elbows bent and hands up by the chest, elbows bent, palms facing forward.

2   Raise your body up by straightening the arms, keeping your body perfectly straight. By bending your elbows lower your chest toward the floor.

Hints & Tips

- Place a soft object below your chest and use it as a marker so that you know you are lowering far enough on each repetition. But make sure it is soft just in case your muscles fatigue.

- To make the exercise harder, try going to a Three-Point Press. To do this bring one foot in to the middle and place the other toe on top of its heel so that they are stacked. This gives you less points of contact so that the muscles have to work harder to lift your weight, (even your abdominals) and you also have to work harder to balance.

Technique

- Lots of other muscles are working hard to support and stabilize your body in this position so keep everything tight—especially your abdominal muscles.

- Always look at the floor rather than up, to keep your spine in neutral alignment.

- Your hands should be level with your chest throughout the exercise. Keep the whole body fixed in that one position.

- When you bend the elbows lower the whole body, not just the chest. Your body should be straight from your shoulders to your heels. No waving your butt in the air!

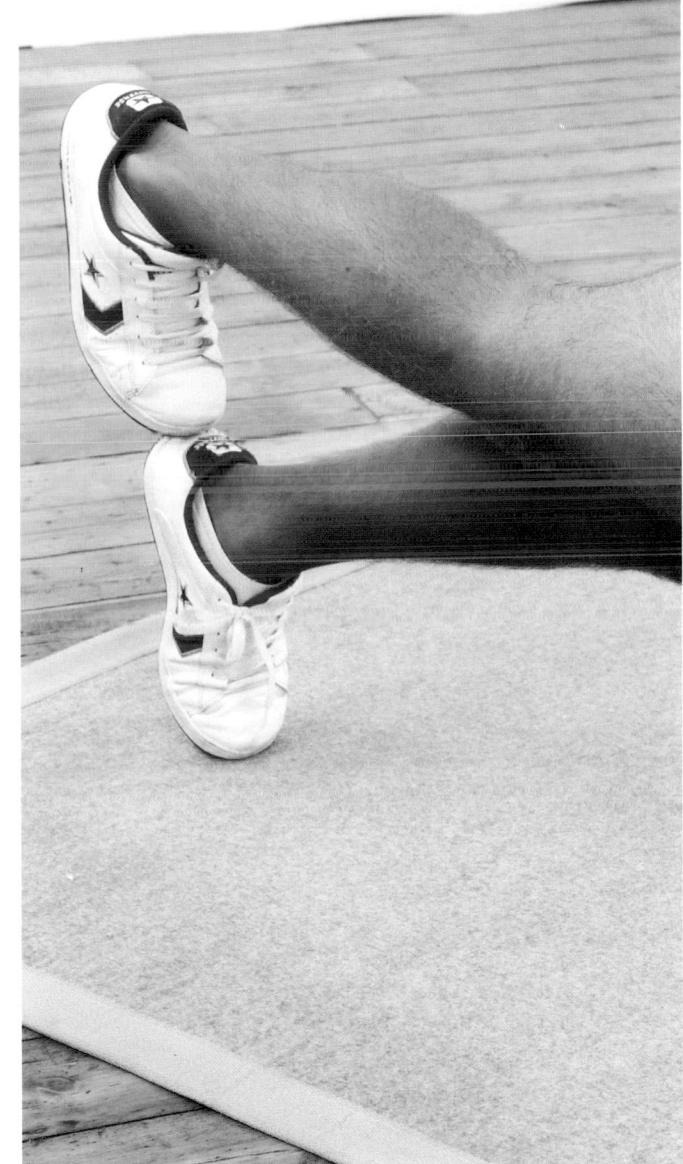

3 The Three-Point Press makes life harder, demanding more tension in the muscles to preserve balance.

Chest—Advanced

decline press up

Area Worked: Upper chest, front of shoulders, and back of arms.
Name of Muscles: Pectoralis, Anterior Deltoid, and Triceps (Abdominal stabilizing).

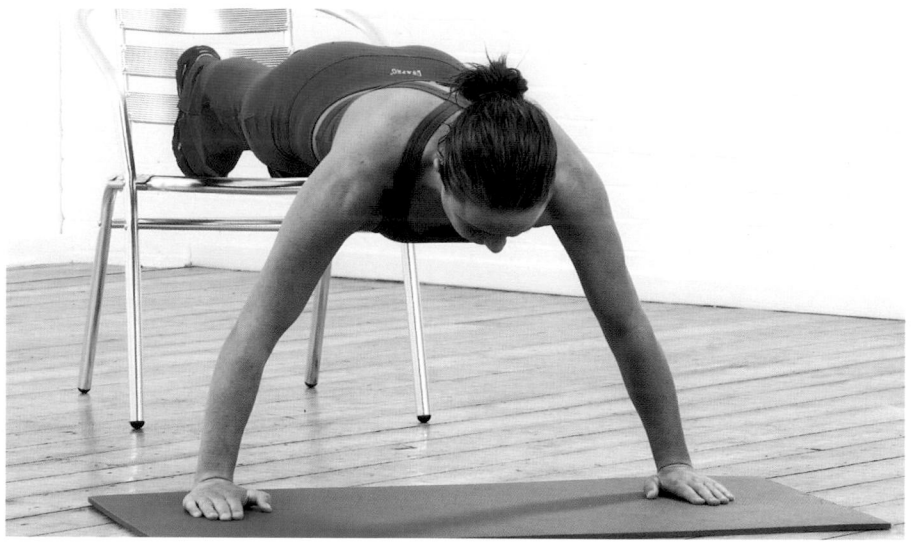

1 Place your feet in an elevated position so that they are raised higher than the rest of your body. They can be placed on a step, chair, or bench, for example.

Hints & Tips

- It becomes very tempting in this exercise to allow the hips to drop. If you let this happen you will usually feel some discomfort in your lower back. Focus on keeping your abdominal muscles braced and tight. If they fatigue and you can no longer maintain a flat back, then rest and try again, rather than risk injury to your back for the sake of a few extra repetitions.

Technique

• By raising your feet higher you now change the emphasis of work onto the upper chest and the shoulders.

• More weight will now be on your arms, so the exercise itself will feel harder.

• Again, like the other styles of Press Up, keep the rest of the body fixed in position and maintain soft elbows.

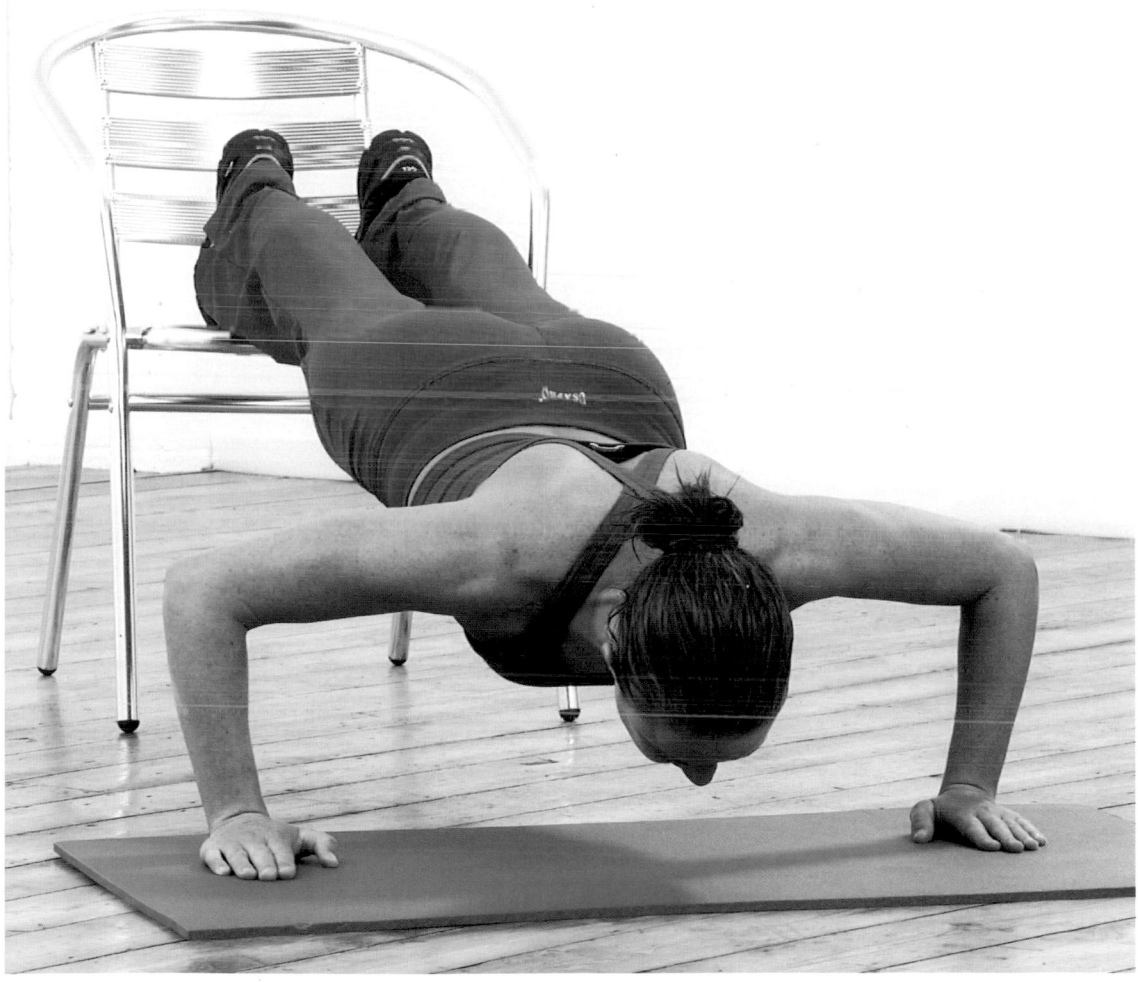

2 Keeping the hands level with the chest, lower your body toward the floor, then push and straighten the arms to return back to the starting position.

Chest–Advanced

dumbbell press up

Area Worked: Chest, front of shoulders, and back of arms.
Name of Muscles: Pectoralis, Anterior Deltoid, and Triceps (Abdominal stabilizing).

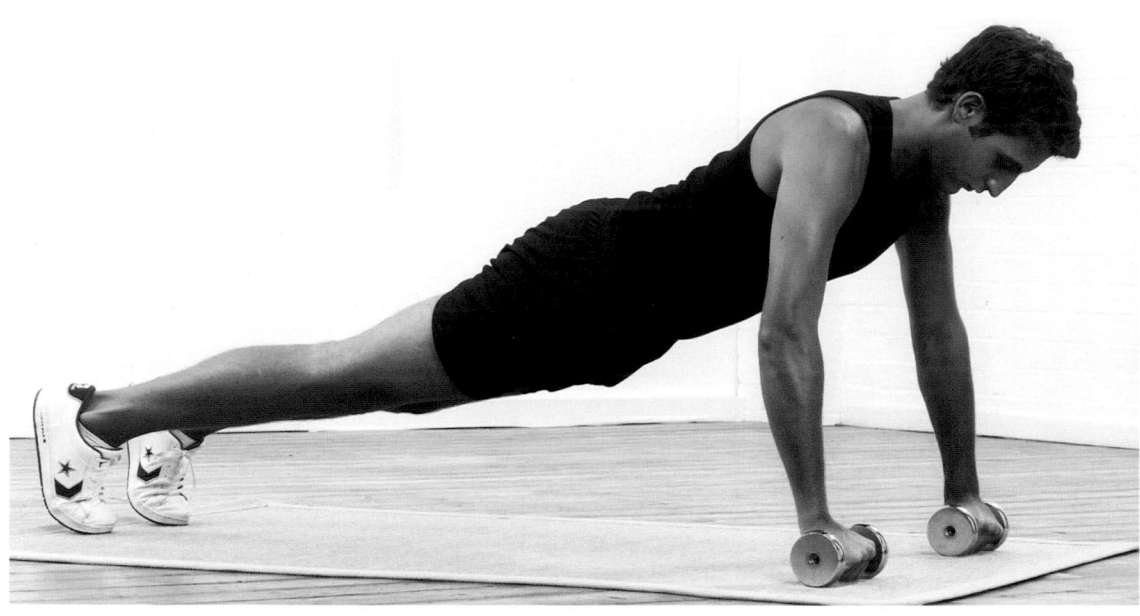

1 Take the standard Full Press Up position (page 36), supporting your weight on your hands and your toes. Now grip the dumbbells and position them where your hands were.

Hints & Tips

- Have the dumbbells ready nearby, or in your hands. Some people find it easier to get in to position with their knees on the floor, then hold the dumbbells and lift the knees. Others are quite happy to grab them and get straight in to the full position. Have a try and find the way that works best for you.

Technique

- The dumbbells are going to destabilize you, which means if you push against them slightly out of line they will move. This means you will have to work harder to stop them moving.

- Keep the movement smooth. The smoother it is, the easier it will be to keep the dumbbells in place. You will soon find out that jerky movements make life harder.

- Keep your knuckles at 90 degrees the floor. This helps to keep the strain off your wrists.

- Because the dumbbells have raised you slightly, be careful how low you go. Going too low can put additional strain onto the shoulders. The dumbbells have effectively replaced the floor, so adjust your depth accordingly.

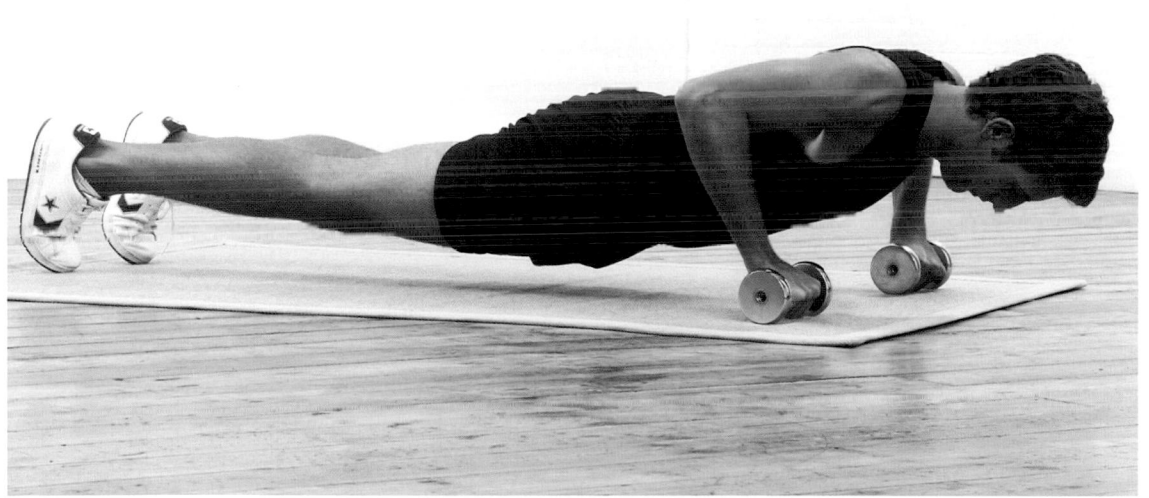

2 Keep your hands and the dumbbells level with your chest and bend the elbows to lower yourself toward the floor. Push against the dumbbells, straightening the arms to return to the start position.

Back–Beginners

single arm dumbbell row

Area Worked: Back, and front of arms.
Name of Muscles: Latissimus Dorsi, and Biceps.

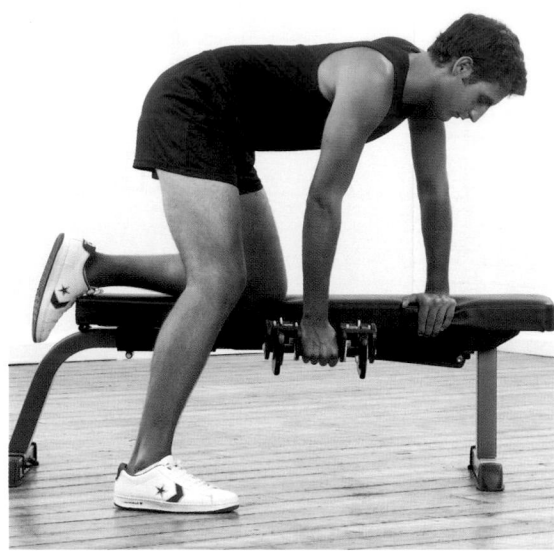 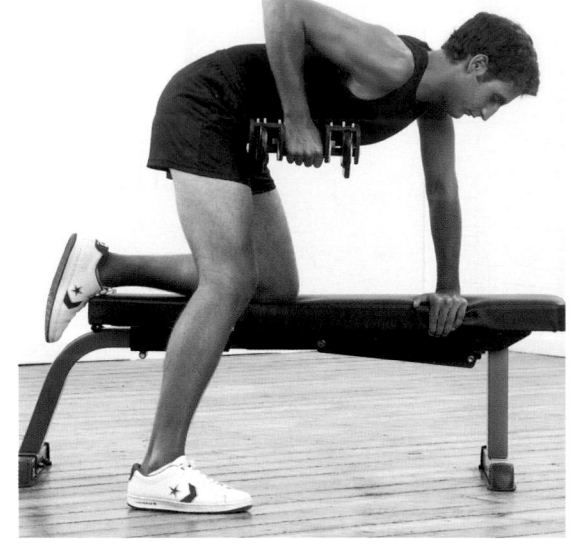

1 Place one hand on a surface that allows you to tip forward so that your back is horizontal. Place the opposite leg slightly wider than your hips.

2 Your arm and feet should make a triangle. Holding the weight at arm's length with the free hand, pull the weight up toward your ribs.

Hints & Tips

- Try to keep your grip and forearms relaxed to emphasize the use of your back muscles. Try to forget about the weight in your hand and concentrate on lifting from your elbow. You naturally want to pull your hand up, which recruits the bicep.

- You should feel the exercise more in your back than your biceps; but this takes practice.

Technique

- Posture is very important during this exercise. Keep the knees soft, hips pushed back, the abdominal muscles pulled in, and keep looking at the floor to maintain the correct position for your back.

- Try not to twist when lifting and lowering the weight. Keep the shoulders parallel with the floor throughout.

- Keep the elbow tucked in to your side as you lift and lower the weight.

- Your elbow should be lifted as high as possible without twisting your body.

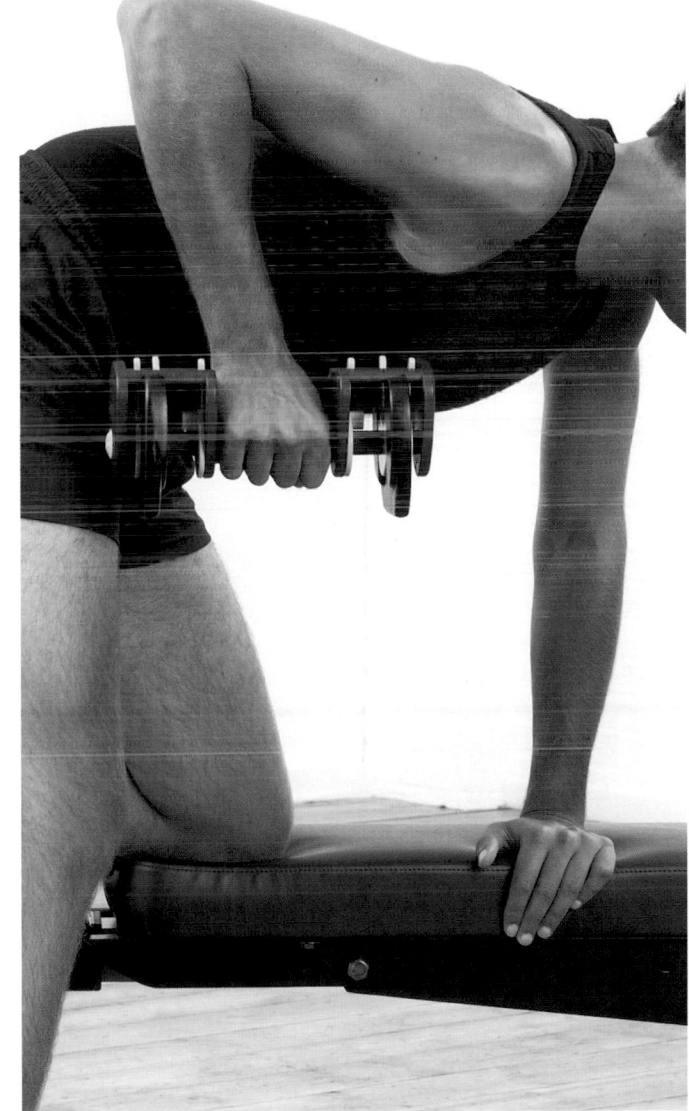

3 Pause for a second before lowering the weight back down. The shoulders are still parallel to the floor at the top of the movement.

Back–Beginners

towel pulldown

Area Worked: Back and Biceps.
Name of Muscles: Latissimus Dorsi and Biceps.

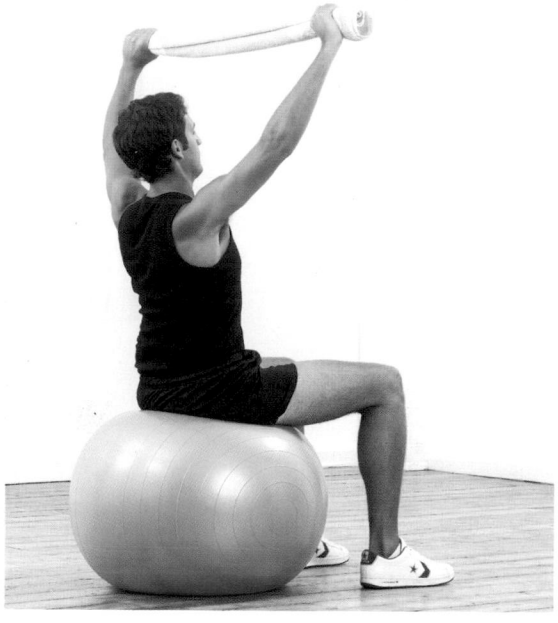

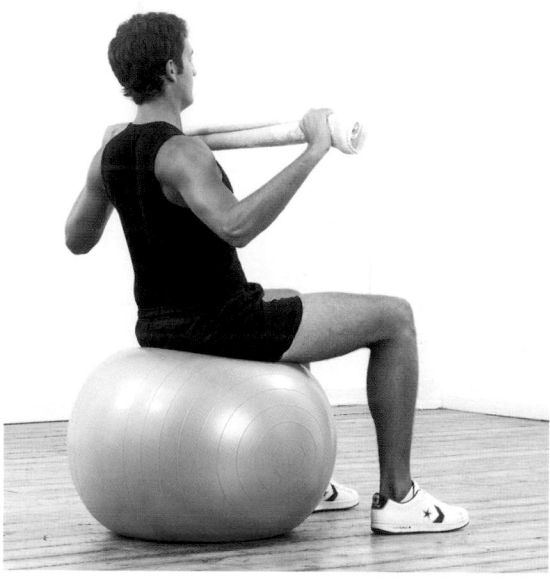

1 Sit on a chair with the towel overhead. Hold the towel so that your body and arms make a "Y" shape.

2 Tilt back slightly and maintain that position. Bending the elbows, pull the towel down to the top of the chest.

Hints & Tips

• The movement from top to bottom should be a straight line from just in front of you to the top of your chest. It is tempting to pull the towel down lower but you do not need to. Focus on that line and remember to maintain your posture at all times. Sit tall!

Technique

- Sit tall on the chair. Pull in the abs, lift the chest and draw the shoulders back. Think good posture.

- When you tilt back do not arch your back but maintain your posture and move from your hips, not your lower back.

- As you pull the towel down, also pull the towel out to the sides as if you were trying to stretch it. The harder you pull, the more you make the muscle work.

- Aim to pull the elbows back behind you and squeeze the shoulder blades together for a second at the bottom of the movement.

3 Do not go down farther than this. Follow the same line to return to the start position.

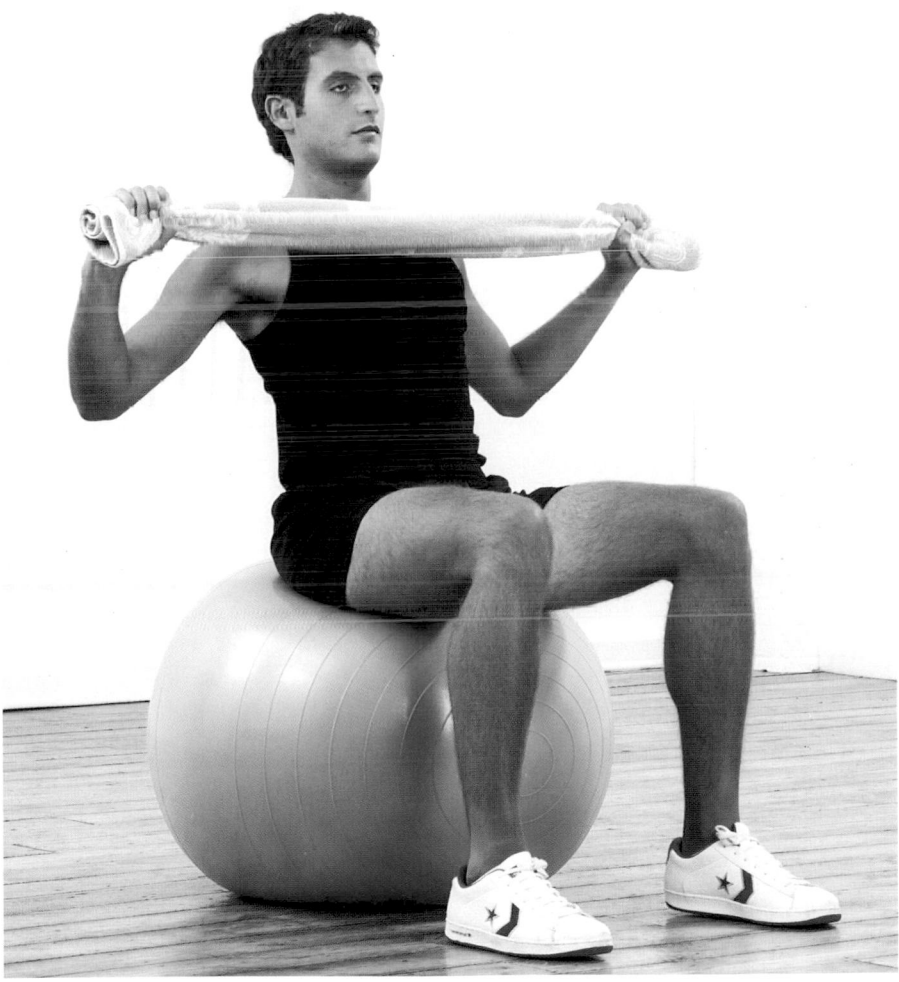

Back—Beginners

shrugs

Area Worked: Upper back.
Name of Muscle: Trapezius.

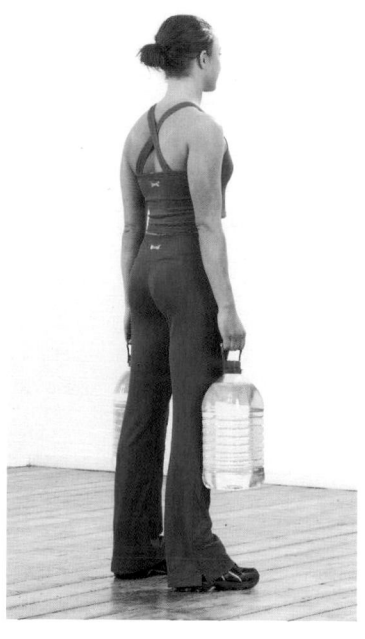

1 Stand up holding a weight in each hand. Focus on your posture so that you have the knees soft, abdominal muscles braced, chest lifted, and shoulders set back.

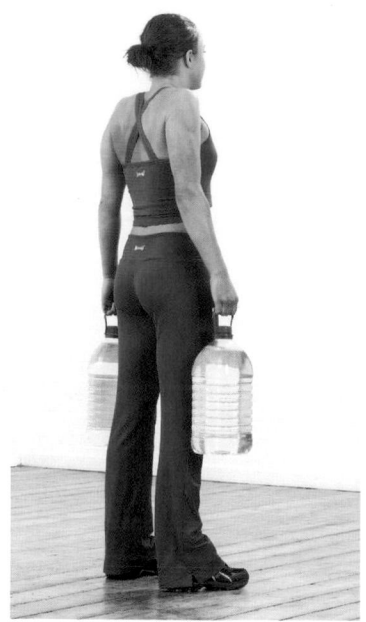

2 Keeping the elbows soft, lift the weights by lifting only your shoulders up toward your ears.

Hints & Tips

- This isn't the most exciting exercise in the world, nor is it the first part of your body that you would probably think of exercising; but it is an important muscle. It is responsible for moving your shoulders back and up and supporting your neck. So in terms of posture it is a very good muscle to exercise. If it helps to keep neck ache at bay that's a bonus!

- The trapezius is a strong muscle, so don't shy away from lifting weights that you may think are heavy; but again, always build up slowly.

Technique

• Maintain your posture throughout the exercise.

• Fix the bend in your elbows. It is tempting to bend the elbows to lift the weights, rather than lifting your shoulders to do it.

• Hold the position at the top for a second so that you are squeezing the shoulders up as high as you can before lowering them.

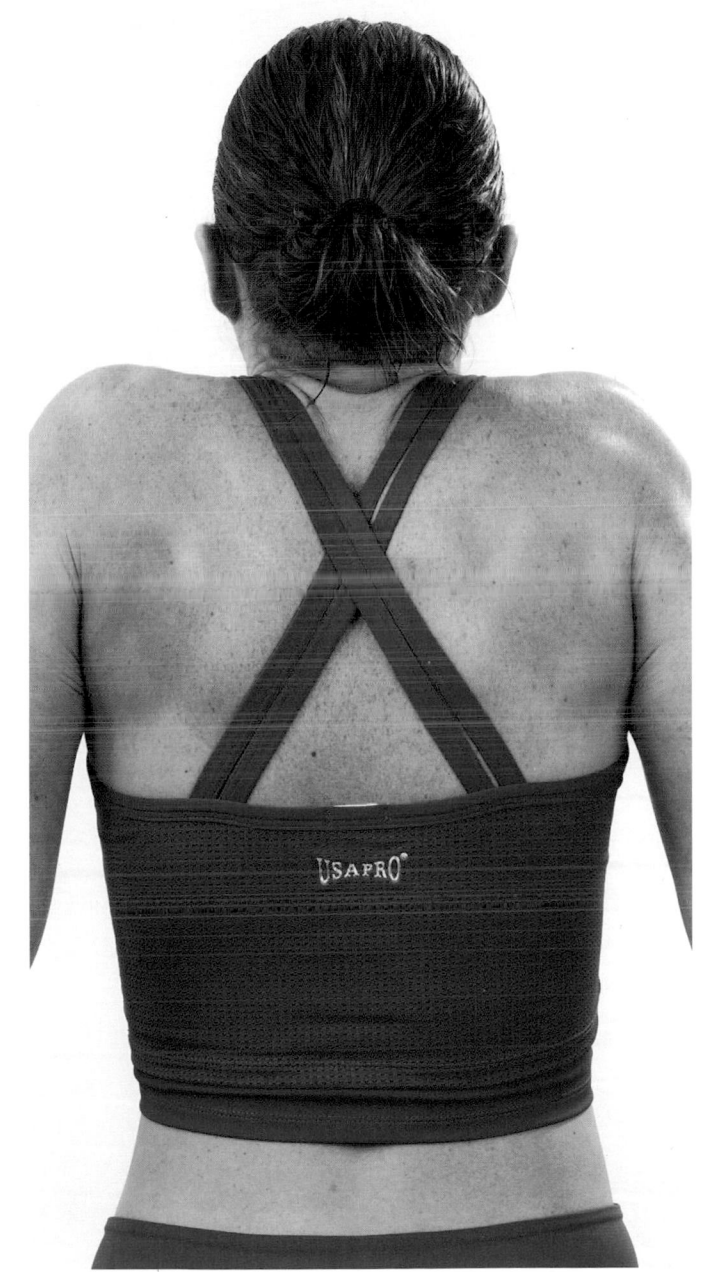

3 Hold for a second at the top of the movement. Lower back down and repeat.

Back–Advanced

bent-over row

Area Worked: Back, and front of arm.
Name of Muscles: Latissimus Dorsi and Biceps.

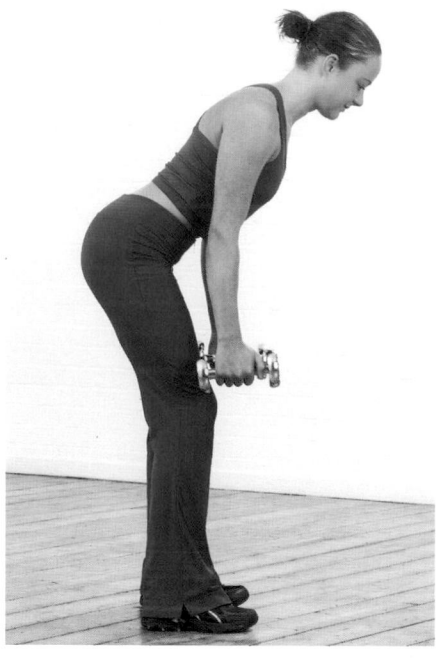
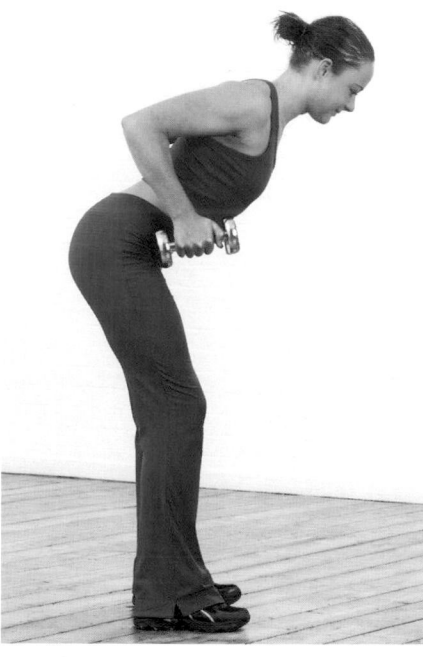

1 Stand tall holding a pair of dumbbells in a neutral grip so that your palms are facing your thighs. Tip forward and let the dumbbells hang down.

2 Your upper body should be at approximately 45 degrees. Pull the dumbbells up into your ribs.

Hints & Tips

• Friends and/or mirrors are handy for checking your posture. Your mid-section should be braced and fixed. The only things that should be moving are your arms lifting the weights.

• To focus more on the muscles in the upper back and backs of the shoulders, go for a wide overhand grip so that your elbows go out and you are pulling the weights up to the sides, level with your chest.

Technique

- Keep the knees soft at all times throughout the exercise.

- Tip from the hips. Keep the head up, lift the chest, pull the abdominal muscles in, and push your hips back as you tip forward. Be very careful not to round your back. It should stay flat.

- Focus on pulling the elbows up past the ribs and keep them tucked in. Pull the shoulders back and squeeze the shoulder blades for a second at the top of the movement before lowering the weights back down.

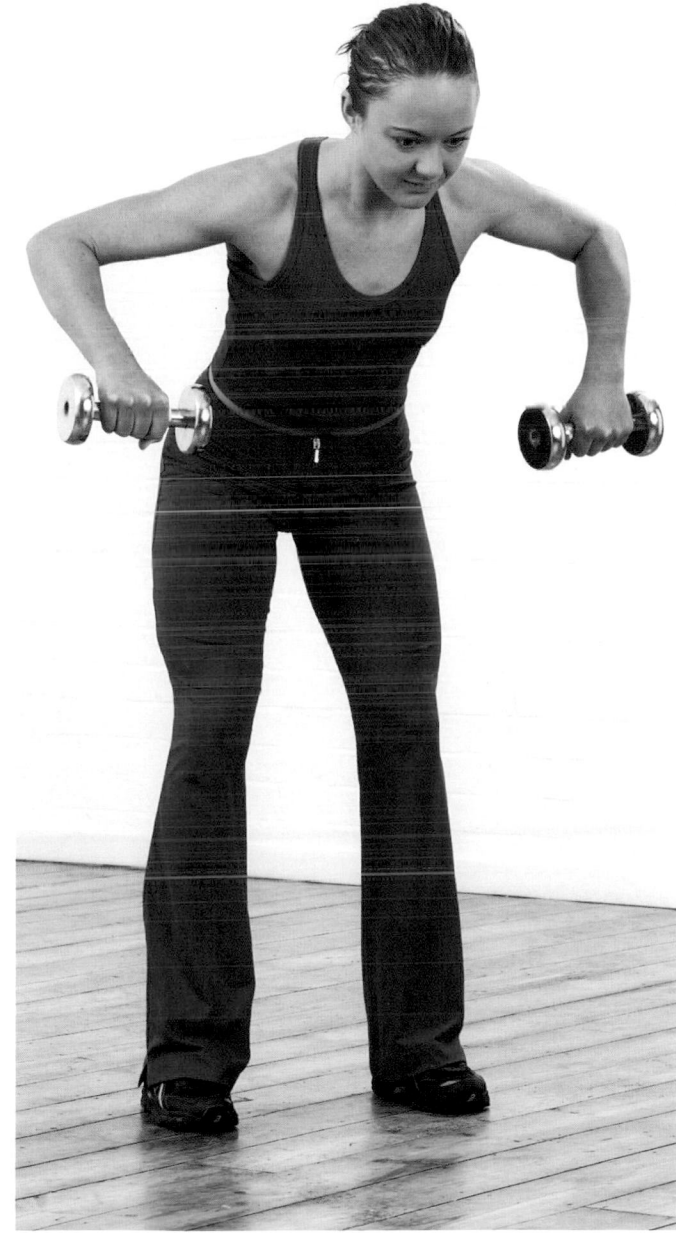

3 The upper back and shoulders are worked more by keeping the hands wider apart.

Back—Advanced

pullover

Area Worked: Back, chest, back of arms.
Name of Muscles: Latissimus Dorsi, Pectoralis, and Triceps. (Abdominals stabilizing).

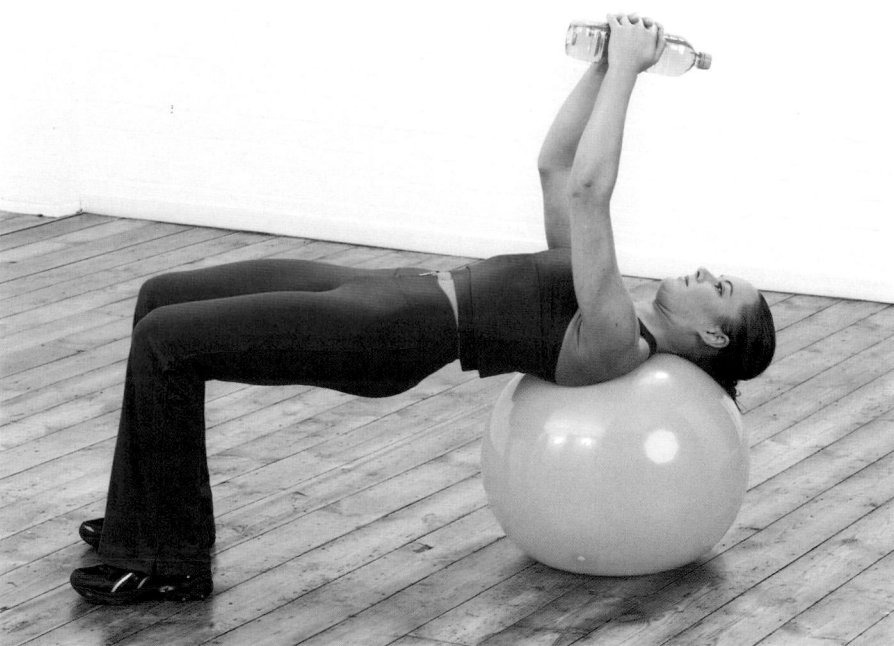

1 Lying on the floor/stability ball or bench hold a weight over your chest. Lower the weight back over the head through a smooth arc.

Hints & Tips

- Find a way to hold the weight that is comfortable for you. Some people cup the weight between thumb and forefinger, while some grip the shaft of the dumbbell.

- You may find that you pull more with one arm than the other depending on how you hold the weight. Either swap the hands over halfway through the set, or practice pulling with both arms equally. The latter would be the better option if you can do it.

Technique

- Keep the abdominal muscles braced throughout the movement. Because you are lowering a weight over the back of your head your back will naturally want to arch. It is up to you and your abdominals to stop this from happening.

- When lowering the weight, put a slight bend in your elbows and keep them fixed in that position.

- Keep the elbows tucked in as if you were squeezing them together.

- You should lower the weight until your arms are approximately parallel with the floor.

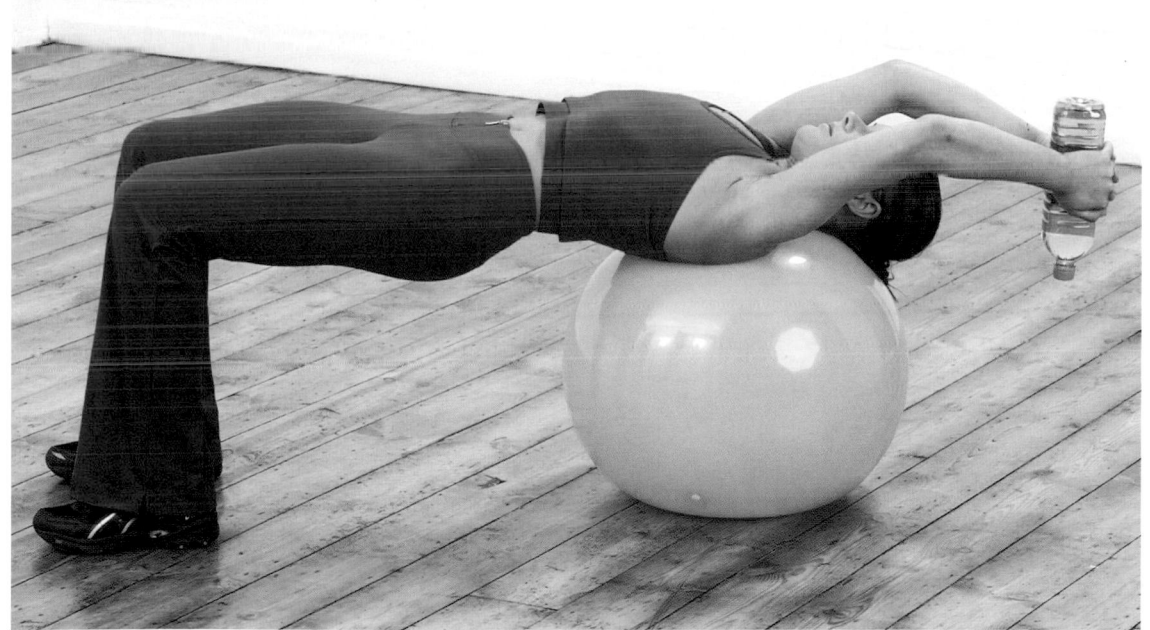

2 Pull the weight back through the same range of movement until it is over your chest.

Back—Advanced

reverse fly

Area Worked: Upper back and back of shoulders.
Name of Muscles: Trapezius and Posterior Deltoid.

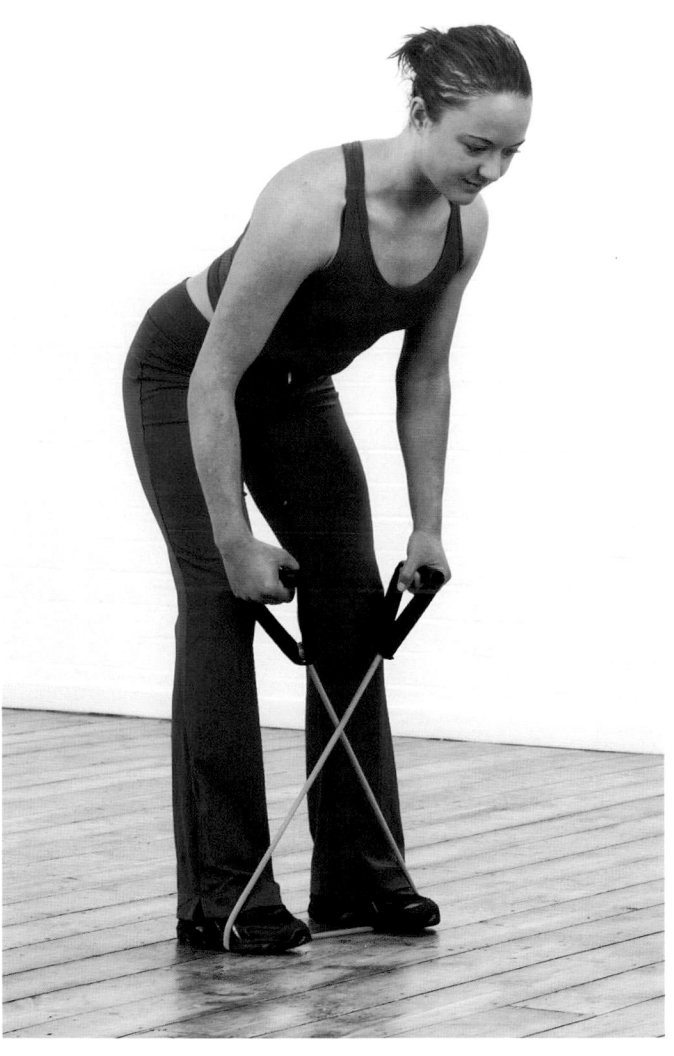

1 Hold a pair of dumbbells (or exercise tube) in a neutral grip so that your palms are facing your thighs. Tip forward so that your upper body is at approximately 45 degrees and let the dumbbells hang down.

Hints & Tips

- Although it may look like you are trying to fly, you aren't, so the speed of movement should reflect this. It should be a slow and controlled lift and a slow and controlled descent.

- Try to keep the muscles under constant tension; do not to let the weights hang at the bottom. Keep those muscles tensed and tight!

- As the exercise gets harder toward the end of the set it becomes tempting to "bounce" the weight up. This usually involves you pushing with your legs and lifting your chest as leverage to get the weights up. Try to maintain good technique even it means putting the weights down and going for the big one next time.

- Start small. You will not need a lot of weight for this one!

Technique

- Keep the knees soft at all times throughout the exercise.

- Tip from the hips. Keep the eyes looking straight ahead, lift the chest, pull the abdominal muscles in, and push your hips back as you tip forward. Be very careful not to round your back. It should stay flat.

- Keep the bend in the elbows fixed throughout the movement. The bigger the bend, the easier the exercise, so it should only be a softening of the joint.

- The range of movement will be determined by the range of movement through your shoulder joints. Make sure each repetition is going as far as you can take it. Remember to squeeze the shoulder blades at the top of each repetition.

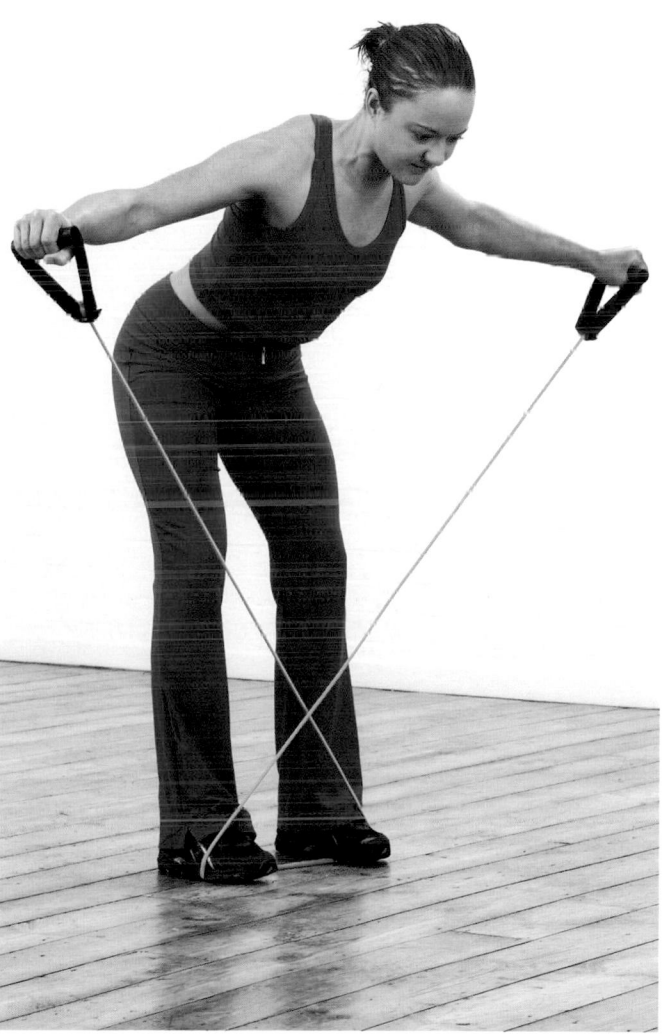

2 Place a slight bend in the elbows. Pull the weights out to the side in a smooth arc until they are as high as they can go. Slowly lower the weights back to their starting position through the same range of movement.

Legs—Beginners

sit down squat

Area Worked: Thighs, butt, and lower back.
Name of Muscles: Quadriceps, Hamstrings, Gluteus, and Erector Spinae.

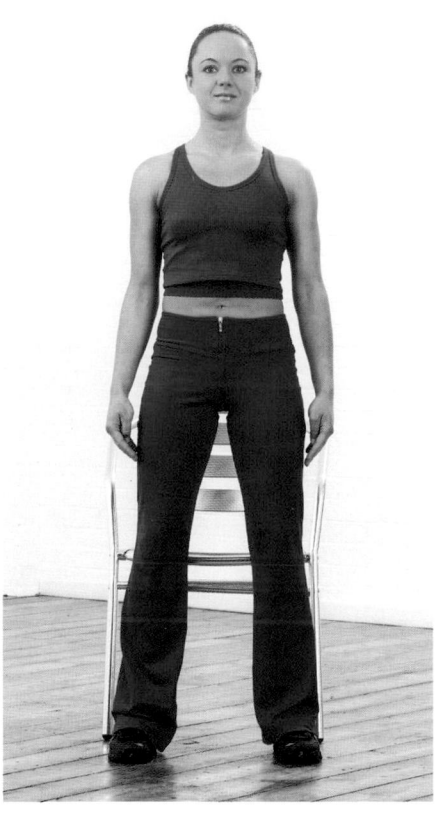
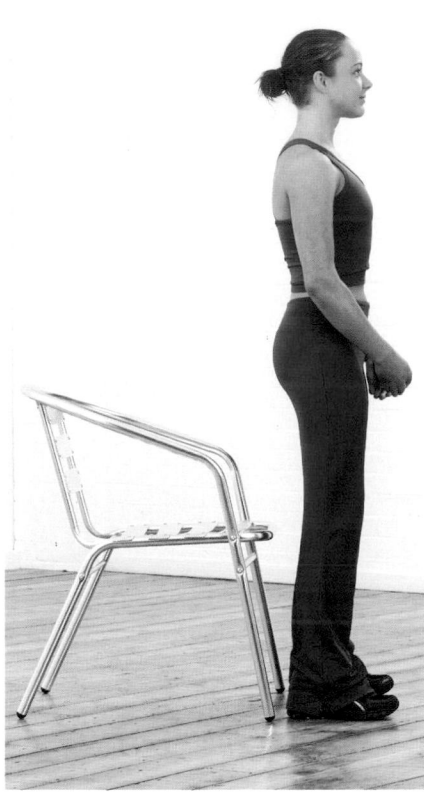

1 and 2 Stand in front of a chair or bench with your back to it. Push the hips back and bend the knees so that you lower yourself down onto the chair or bench.

Hints & Tips

• When squatting, always look straight ahead. If you look down, the rest of your back will want to follow, which means that it is likely that your lower back will round. This could lead to injury.

Technique

- The chair or bench should be of such a height that when you fully sit onto it your knees are at approximately 90 degrees and your thighs are parallel with the floor.

- Focus on pushing the hips back before you start to bend the knees. Keep the chest lifted and look straight ahead to keep your spine in a neutral position.

- You should sit, but still holding your position. Do not fully relax on the seat.

- Try to do most of the pushing with your heels when straightening back up and remember to stand tall at the top of the movement.

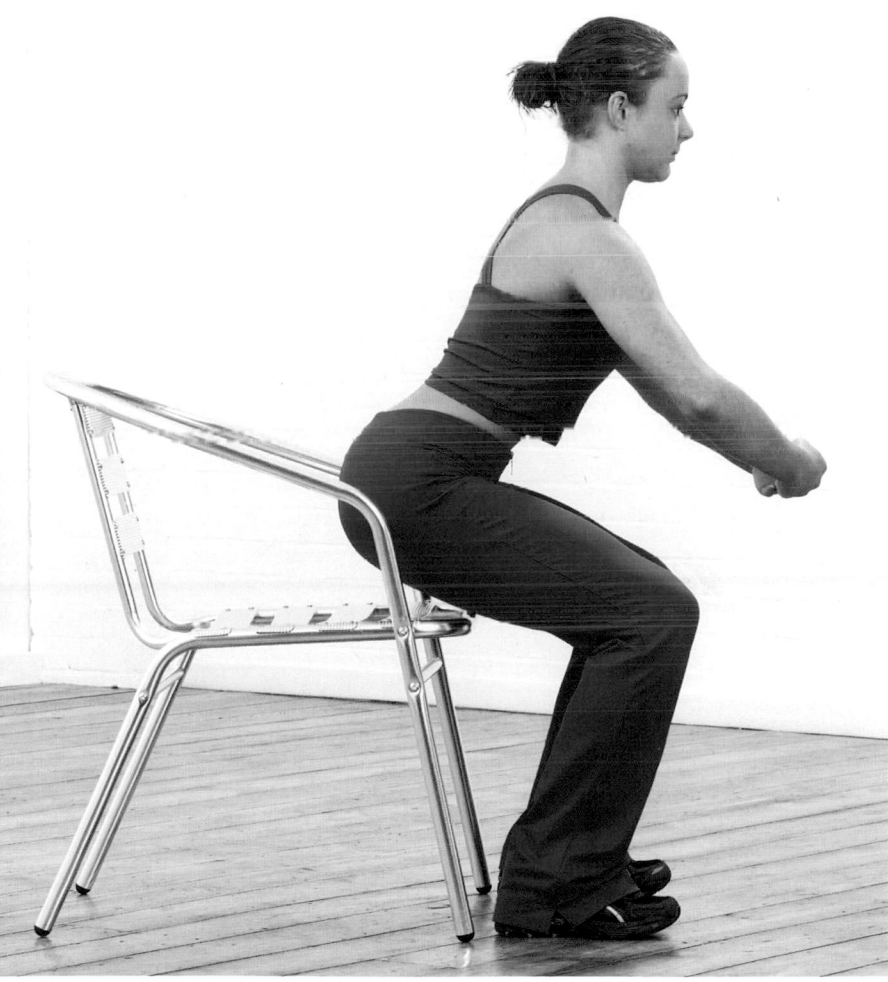

3 Sit lightly and pause for a moment, with the leg muscles still working, before standing up again.

Legs–Beginners
lunge

Area Worked: Thighs and butt.
Name of Muscles: Quadriceps, Hamstrings, and Gluteus.

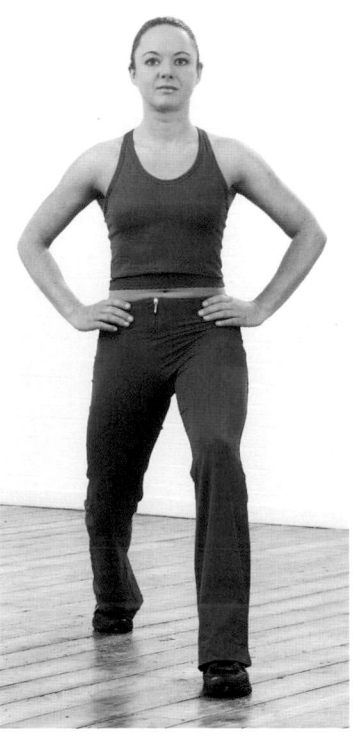

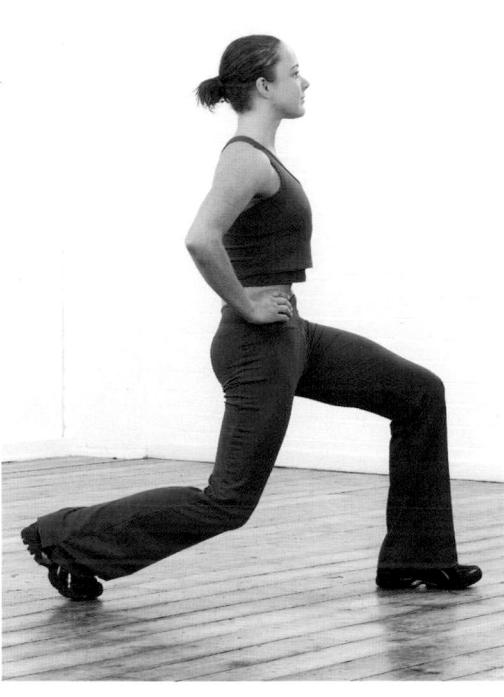

1 Stand tall with your feet hip-width apart.

2 Take a big step forward and raise the heel of your back foot. Keeping the body upright, bend the knees and lower down toward the floor.

Hints & Tips

• Try to visualize two parallel lines projecting forward from your feet so that when you step forward your feet stay on the same lines.

• To maintain an upright position, focus on lifting the chest and drawing the shoulders back.

Technique

• Maintain the upright position of your body throughout the exercise. Try not to lean forward.

• When stepping forward maintain hip-width position with the feet. It is very easy to bring them closer together when you step.

• Lower down slowly and be careful that you don't hit your knee on the floor.

• Focus on pushing through the heel of the front foot and the toe of the back foot.

• Avoid locking the knees as you come up.

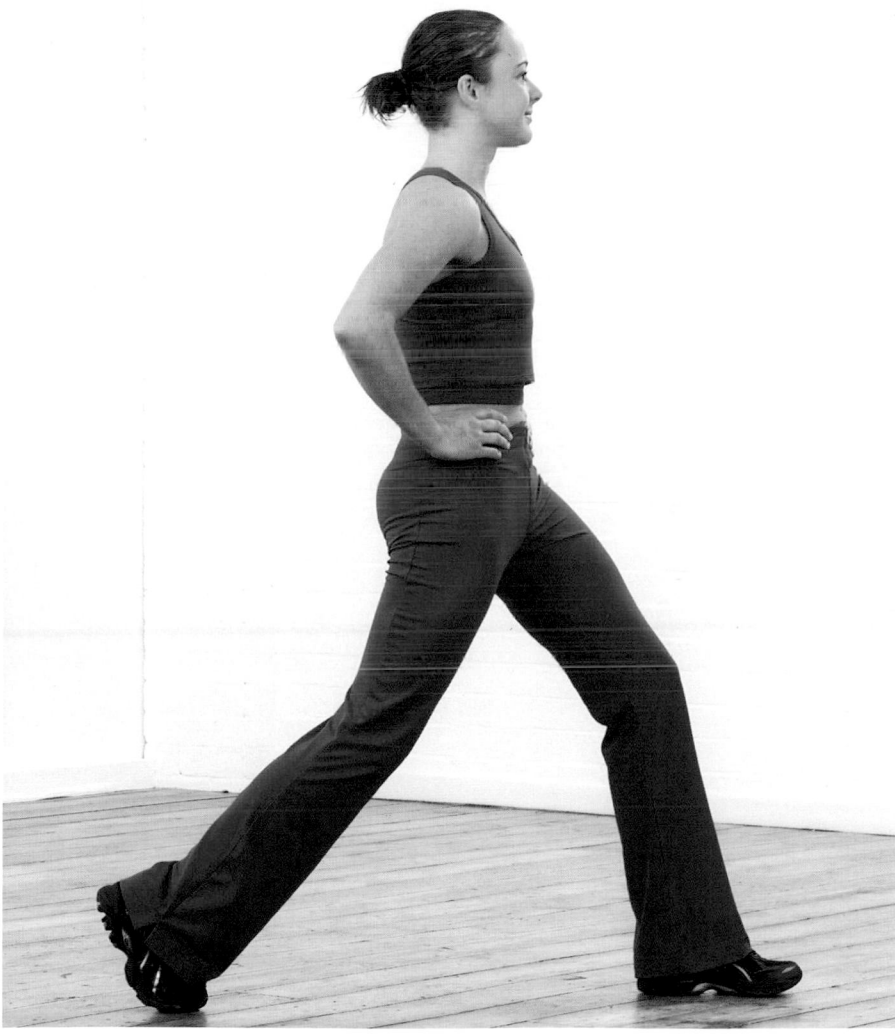

3 Push into the floor and straighten the legs again. Repeat for the set number of repetitions. Swap the legs over and do an equal number of repetitions.

Legs—Beginners

calf raise

Area Worked: Back of lower leg.
Name of Muscles: Gastrocnemius and Soleus.

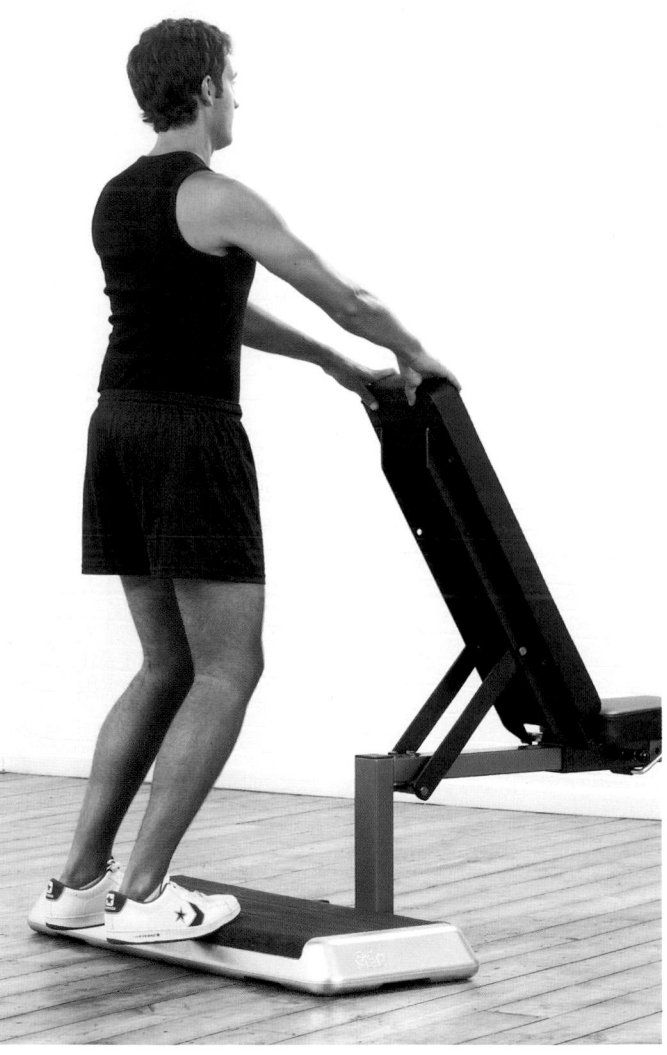

1 Position yourself on a step or stair. Move your feet so that you can pivot on the balls of your feet with your heels of the edge.

Hints & Tips

- Your calves get a lot of work each day so they can lift quite a lot of weight. If you feel you can progress then try the calf raises on one leg at a time.

Technique

• Stand tall throughout the movement. Try to find somewhere to do the exercise where you can lightly hold on to something without compromising your posture.

• Keep the knees straight, but not locked, when lifting and lowering the heels.

• You should feel the muscle stretch as you lower and tighten as you lift.

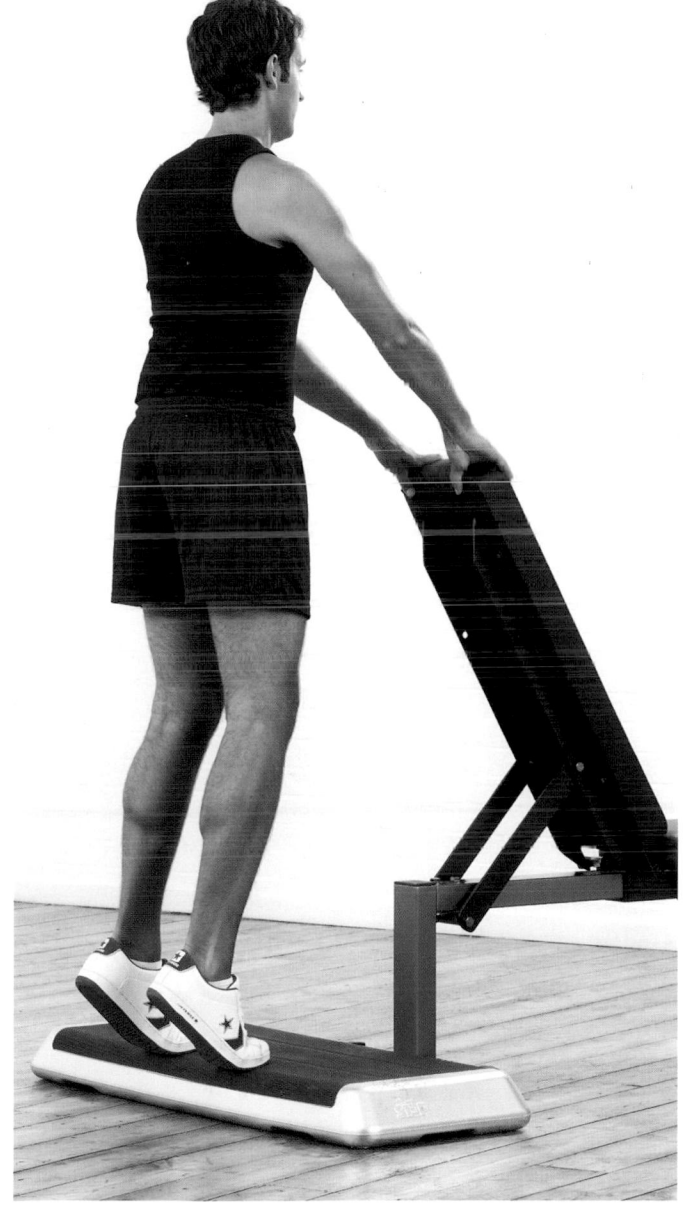

2 While keeping the legs straight, slowly lower the heels down toward the floor and then push your heels up so that you are standing on your toes. Repeat once.

Legs–Beginners

glute raise

Area Worked: Butt.
Name of Muscle: Gluteus.

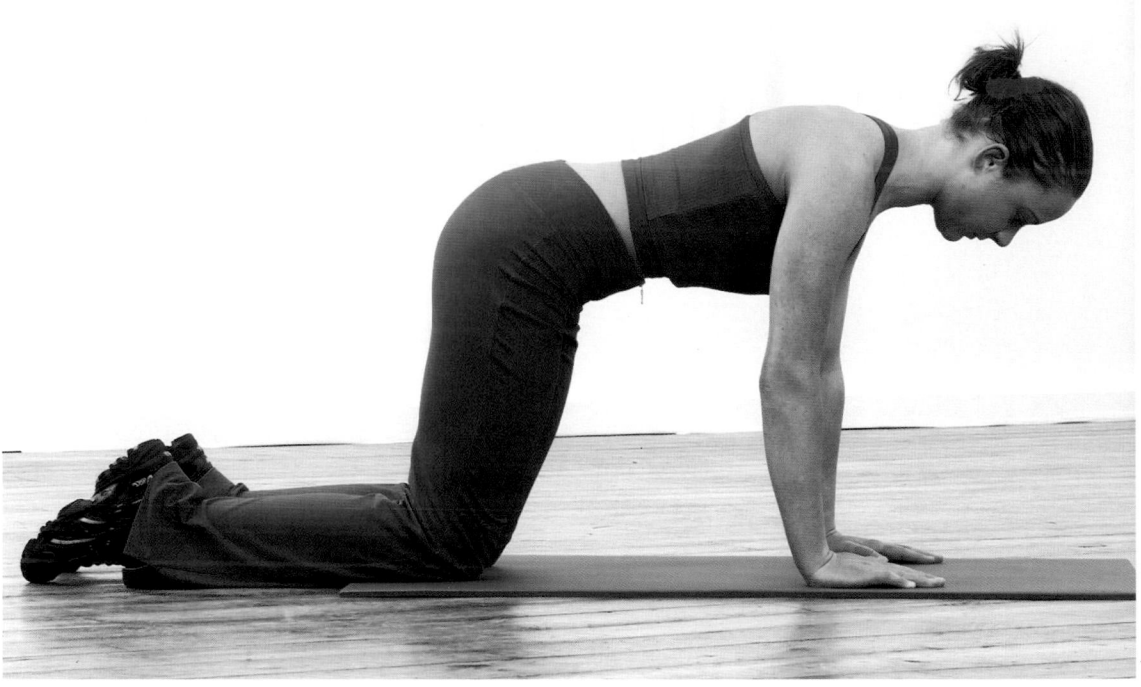

1 Position yourself on all fours on the floor.

Hints & Tips

- You can make the exercise harder or easier by straightening or bending the knee.

Technique

- Keep the elbows soft and directly beneath your shoulders. Keep the abdominal muscles pulled in and your back flat. Always look at the floor.

- Focus on pushing the heel up as high as you can each time without twisting the body.

- Move the heel through an arc rather than straight up and down.

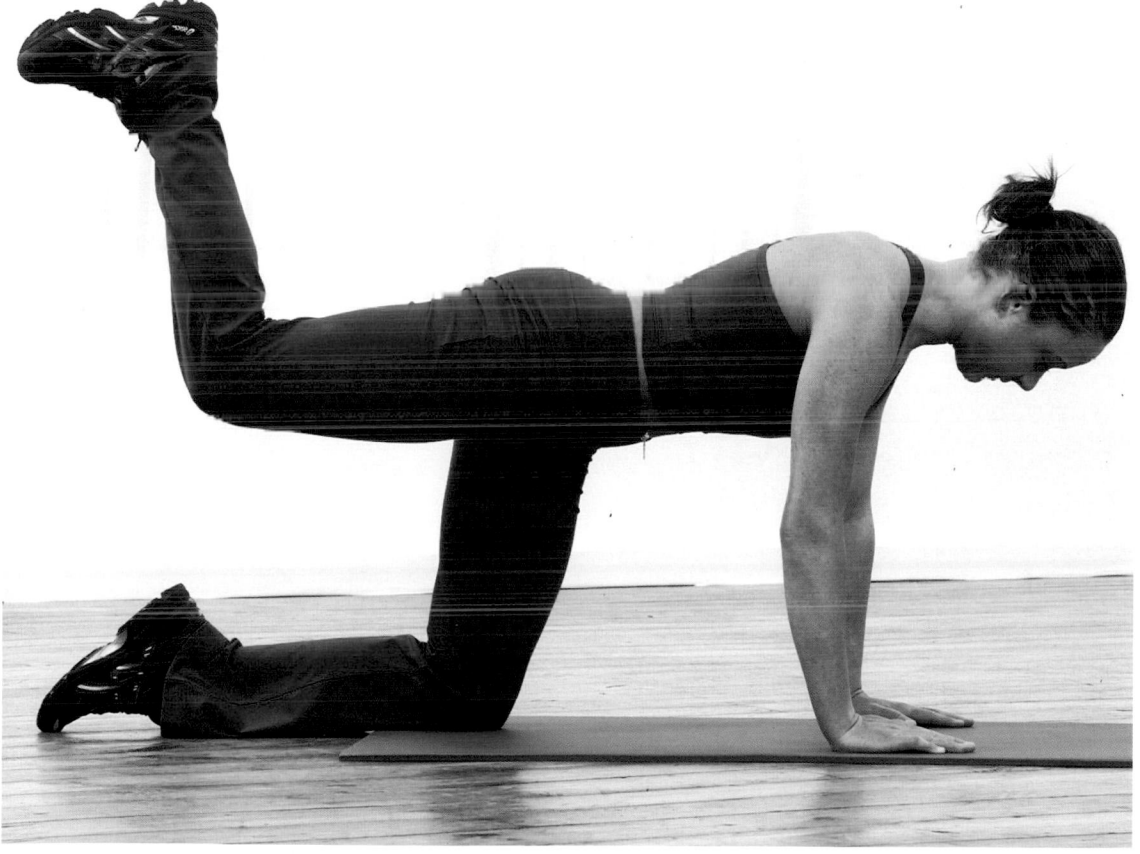

2 Raise one knee off the floor. While keeping the knee bent, push the heel of the foot up toward the ceiling. Slowly lower halfway back down and repeat.

Legs—Advanced

weighted squat

Area Worked: Thighs, butt, and lower back.
Name of Muscles: Quadriceps, Hamstrings, Gluteus, and Erector Spinae.

1 Stand tall, holding a weight in each hand. Push the hips back and bend the knees so that you lower yourself down.

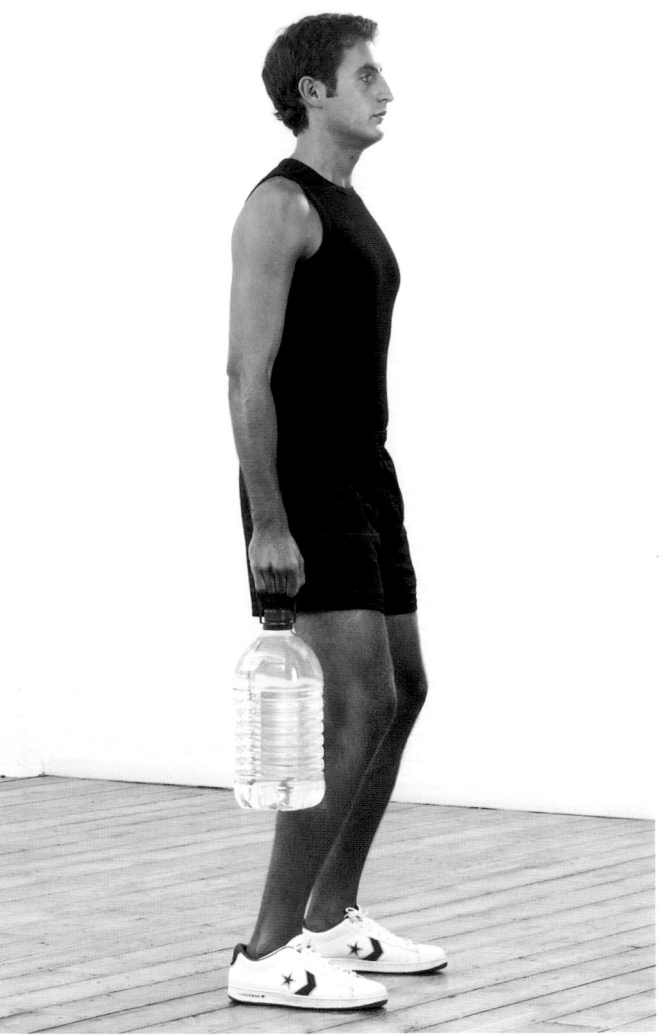

Hints & Tips

- To help practice keeping the weight on your heels and help practice your balance, try this easy drill. Without any weights, lower yourself down into the squat very slowly. As you move down try to lift your toes and the front of your foot very slightly. If you have got the movement right, you should be able to do this and still keep your balance.

Technique

- Keep the feet slightly wider than hip-width throughout the movement.

- Start the movement by tilting the hips back and then follow by bending the knees. Keep looking straight ahead and remember to lift the chest as you lower down. These four points will help you to keep your back straight.

- Your knees should track over your toes. There should be a straight line from your hip, through your knees, and down to your toes.

- Keep the arms straight but not locked. The weights are there purely to add resistance to make the exercises harder.

- At the top of the movement remember to come all the way back up, but keep the knees soft. If you begin to feel tension building in your lower back, you may not be coming back up far enough. Remember to tilt your hips back into their neutral position.

- Try to do most of the pushing (60–70%) through your heels.

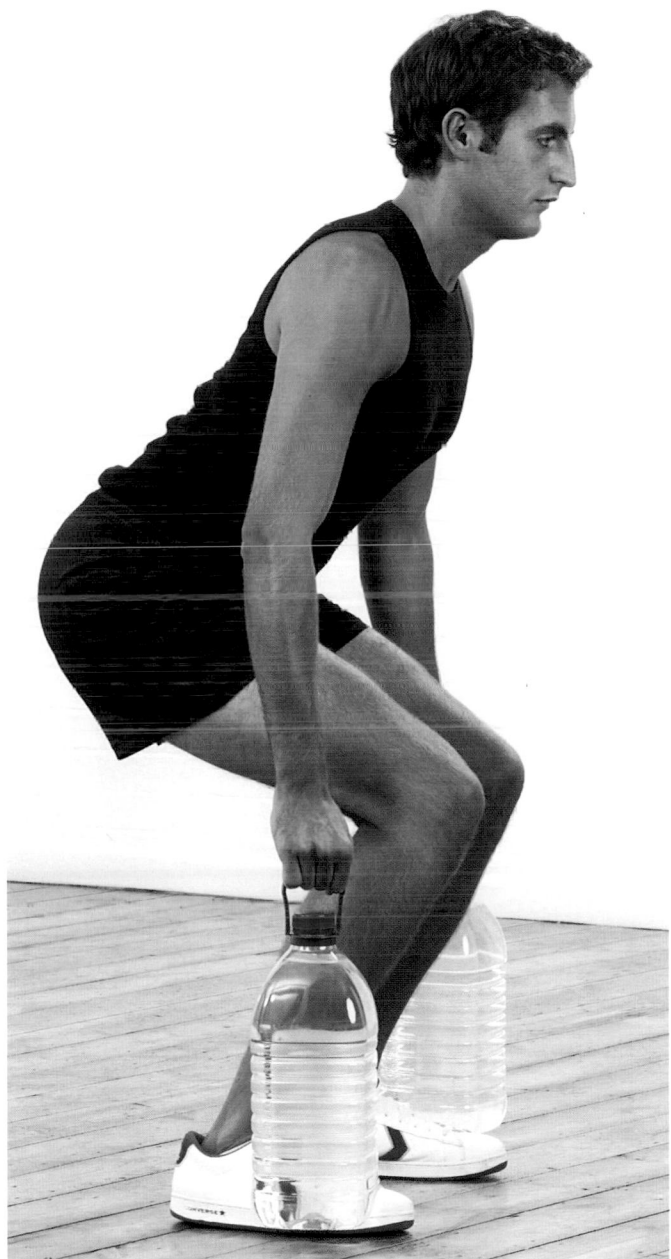

2 When the thighs are approximately parallel to the floor push and straighten the legs to return to the start position.

Legs–Advanced

plié squat

Area Worked: Thighs, butt, and lower back.
Name of Muscles: Quadriceps, Hamstrings, Adductors, Gluteus, and Erector Spinae.

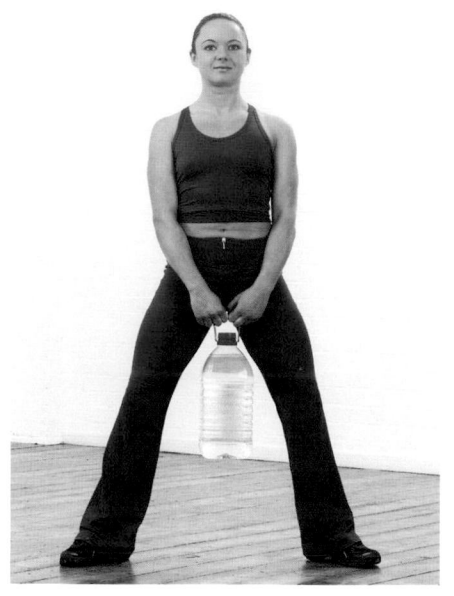

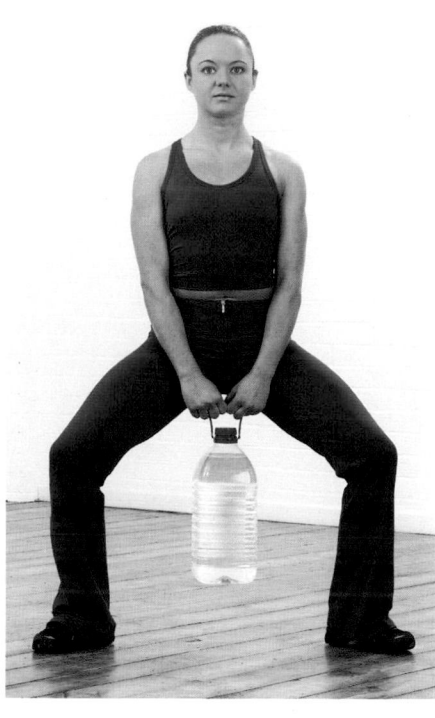

2 The toes should be turned slightly outward. Push the hips back and bend the knees so that you lower yourself down.

1 Stand tall, holding a weight in each hand or a single weight in both hands. Place the feet about one-and-a-half times hip-width.

Hints & Tips

• Because your feet are now wider apart, they may be in the way of your weights as you lower. One way around this is to hold a weight in both hands in front of you as you lower down (as above). Be careful your chest does not fall forward under the weight and round your back. Exaggerate lifting the chest to counter this.

Technique

- The movement itself is identical to the Weighted Squat but helps to target the inner thigh.

- The width of your feet can be varied depending on the individual. The wider your feet go, the more your inner thigh has to work. But remember to check that your knees are tracking over the toes. The wider your feet are the harder this becomes. If you feel strain on the knees joint itself it may be that your feet are too wide.

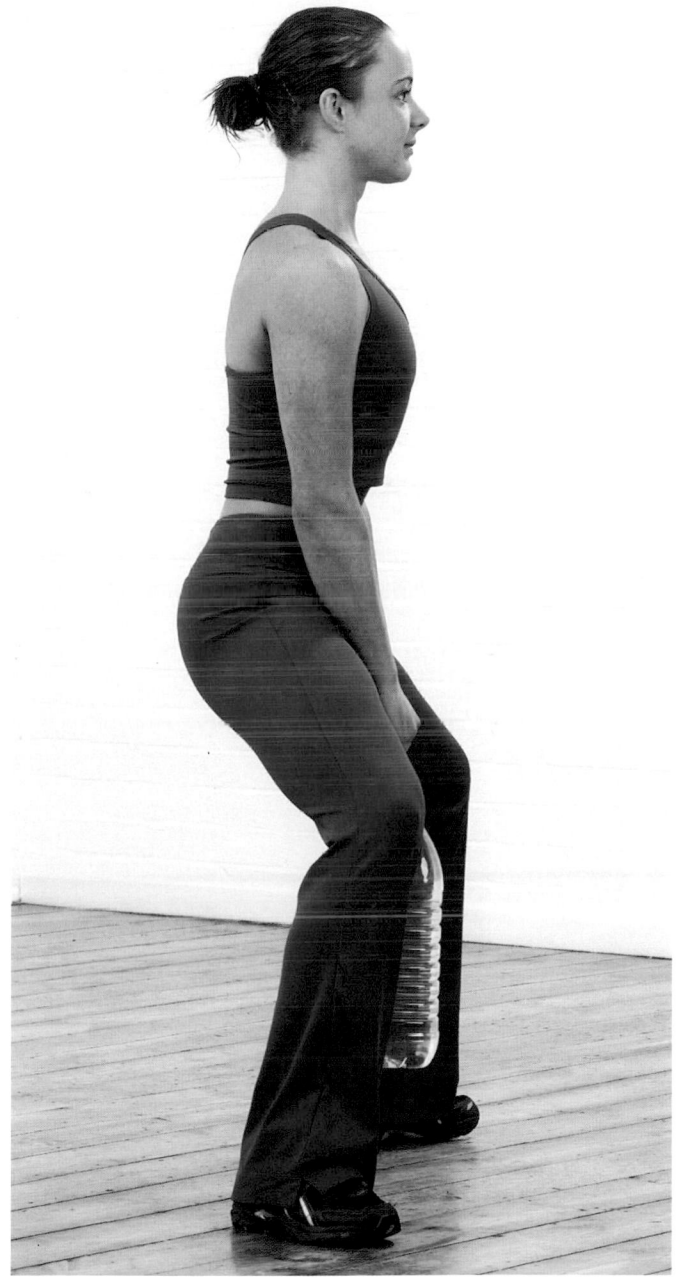

3 When the thighs are approximately parallel to the floor, push and straighten the legs to return to the start position.

Legs—Advanced

Romanian deadlift

Area Worked: Back of thighs, butt, and lower back.
Name of Muscles: Hamstrings, Gluteus, and Erector Spinae.

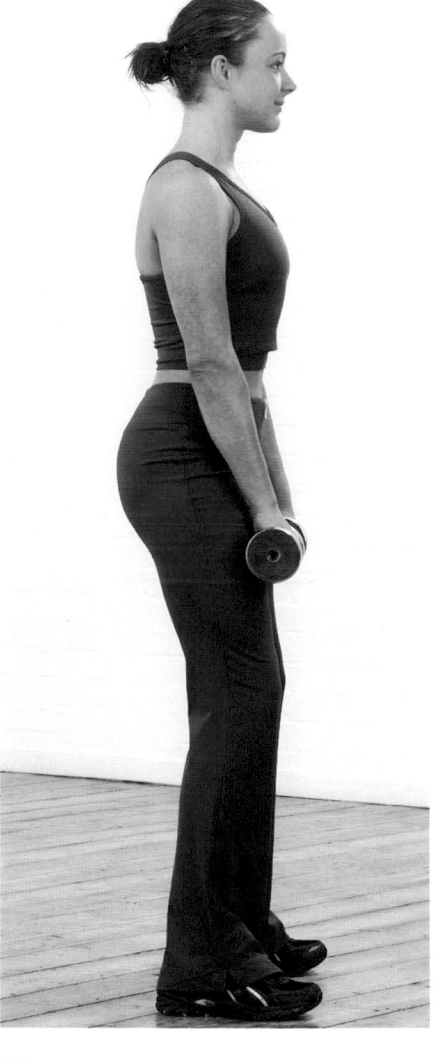

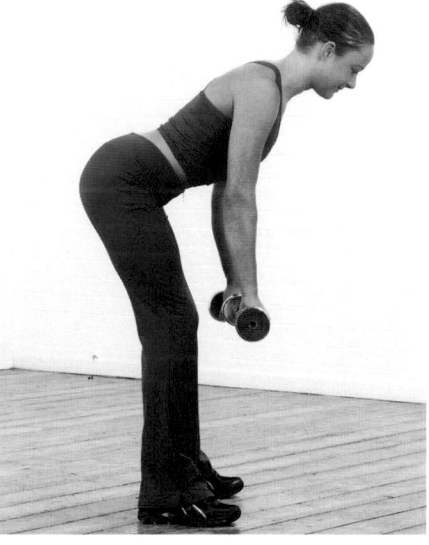

1 Stand tall and hold a weight in each hand, palms inward.

2 Place a slight bend in the knee. Keeping that bend in the knee, push the hips back and tip the upper body forward toward the floor.

Hints & Tips

- Focus on moving from your hip joint and not your back. The back position you adopt in relation to neck and hips, before you start to lower, should be the same position even when you are at the lowest point.

- As a rule of thumb, you are aiming for your hands to be around knee height at the lowest point but this will be dependent on your flexibility.

- Find a mirror, or a friend to check your posture for you. It is hard to tell if you are in the correct position when you are on your own.

Technique

- The feet should be approximately hip-width apart for this exercise.

- You are placing a bend in the knee which goes just beyond "softening" the knee joint. Once you have this position, the angle at your knee should not change.

- Before you start to tip the upper body forward, pull the abdominals in, lift the chest, and push your hips back.

- Maintain this position throughout the lifting and lowering movement.

- You should start to feel a mild stretch down the back of the thighs as you tip forward, but be careful not to go too far as this will cause your back to round.

- Keep the head aligned with the back as you move through the exercise. Try not to look up or down.

- Keep the arms relatively relaxed and allow them to move as you lift and lower. They should just hang and pivot at the shoulder.

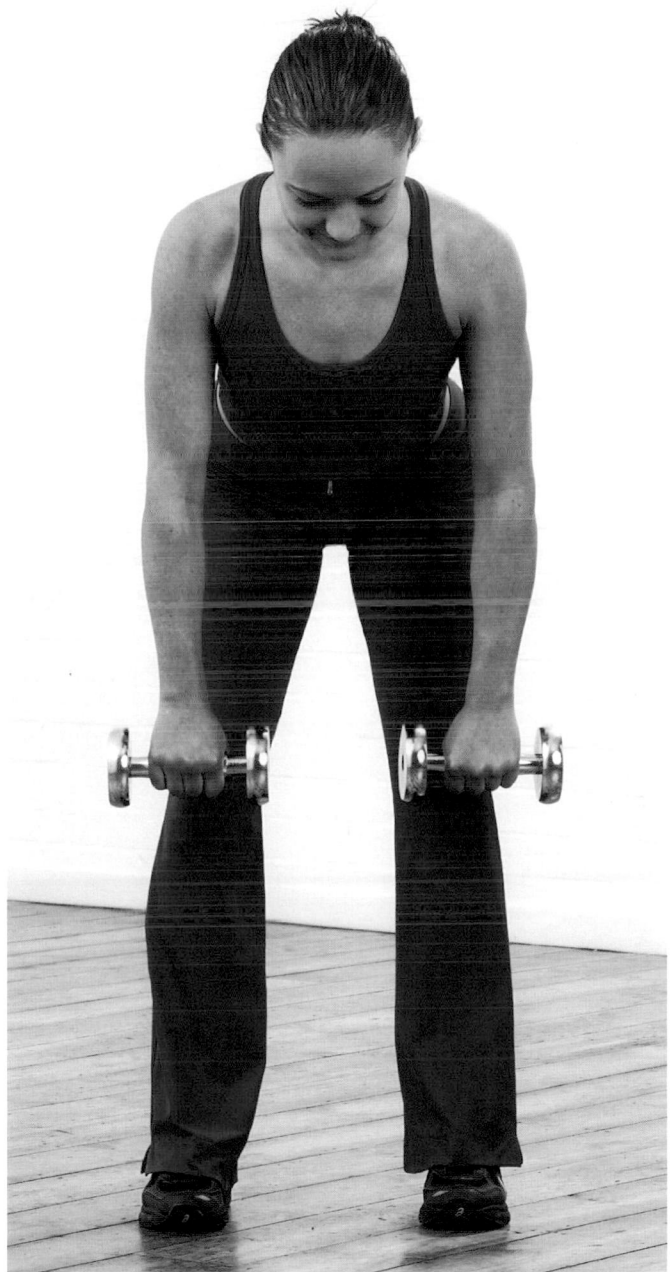

3 Lift the upper body and return to the start position.

Legs—Advanced

power squat

Area Worked: Thighs, butt, lower back, and back of lower leg.
Name of Muscles: Quadriceps, Hamstrings, Gluteus, Erector Spinae, Gastrocnemius, Soleus.

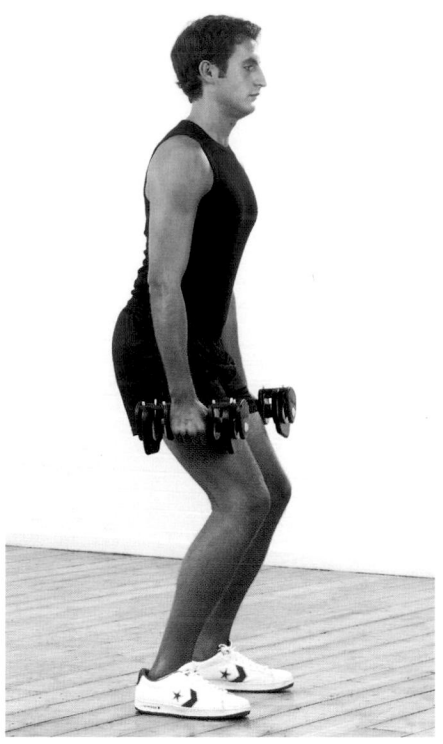 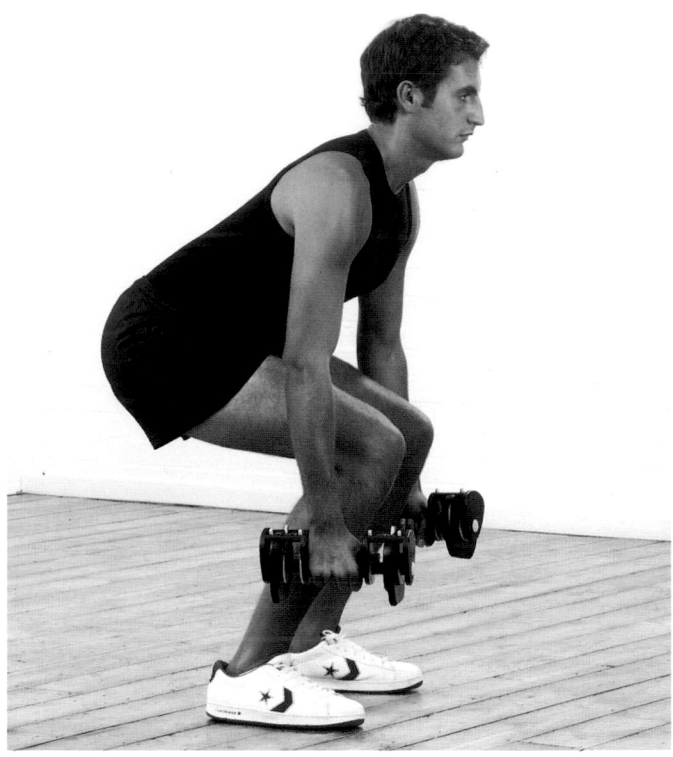

1 Stand tall holding a weight in each hand.

2 Push the hips back and bend the knees to lower yourself down.

Hints & Tips

- Keep the weight slightly lighter then the Weighted Squat initially, until you have become accustomed to the speed of the movement.

Technique

• The Power Squat is very like the Weighted Squat. The only difference is the speed of movement from your lowest point and the subsequent lifting of the heels. It is essentially a combination of the Weighted Squat and the "top half" of the Calf Raise.

• When pushing back up, keep the change of direction smooth and accelerate. Remember to push with your heels.

• When you approach the top of the movement allow your heels to lift with the momentum generated. As they lift, concentrate on your balance and lift the heels as high as you can so that you feel the lower leg tighten up.

• Be careful that you do not lock your knees at the top at the point just before your heels start to lift. Keep them soft.

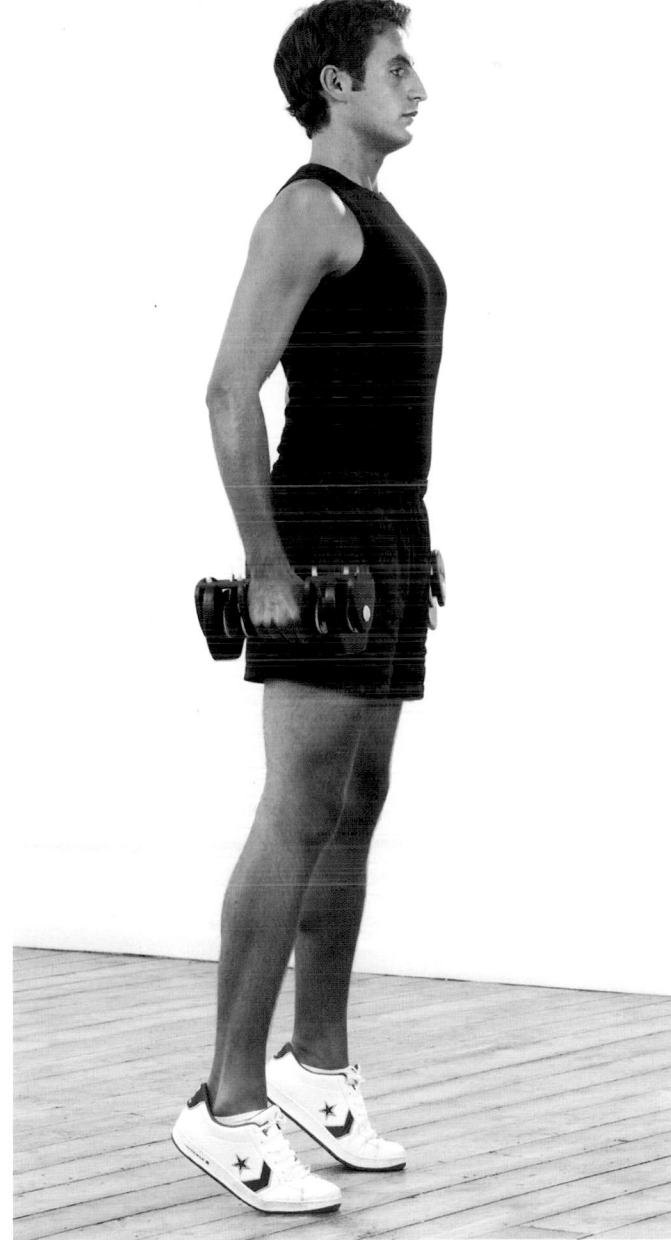

3 Continue to lift the heels until you are on your toes and then lower back down to the start position.

Arms—Beginners

bicep curl

Area Worked: Front of the arms.
Name of Muscles: Biceps.

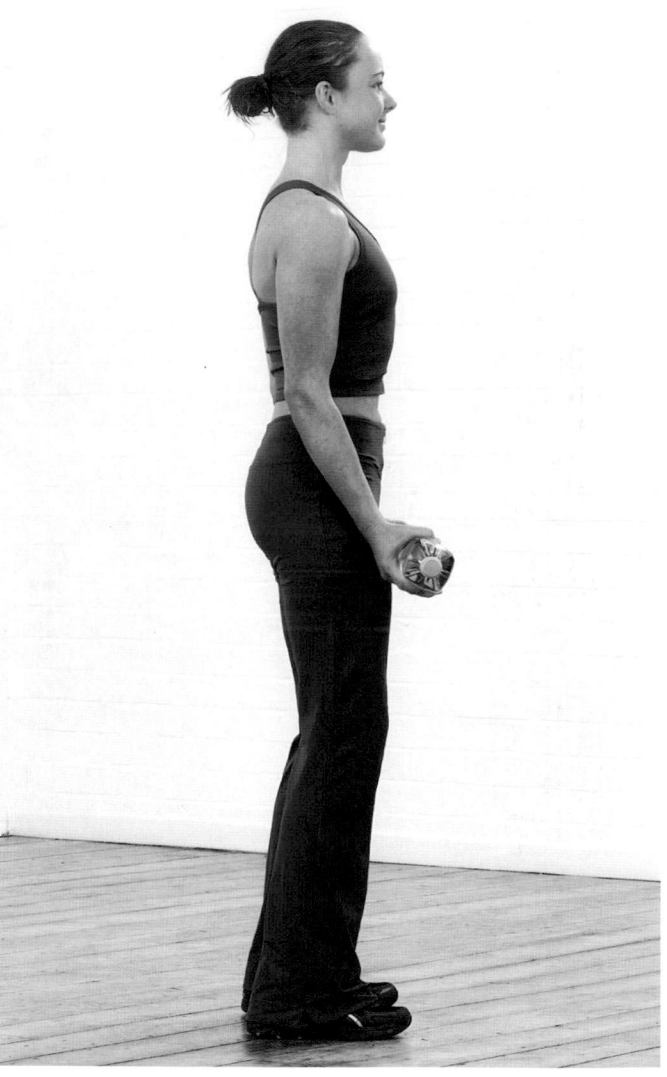

1 Stand tall, holding the weights in your hand so that they are by your thighs. Turn the palms so that they face forward. Bend the elbows and lift the weights up toward your shoulders.

Hints & Tips

- The biggest mistake made on this exercise is swinging the weight up, rather than curling the weight up. Really focus on fixing your elbows. Pin them in to your sides and do not let them move.

- At the top of the movement your hands or the weights should not touch your shoulders. If they do, check the position of your elbows. Are they still in the same place or have they drifted forward?

Technique

- Keep your elbows fixed in that single position by your sides. Your elbows are acting as a hinge, so fix them in place to make the bicep muscle do all the work.

- Do not let your wrists flop down. Keep them straight.

- Keep your mid section braced and do not let the weights pull you forward.

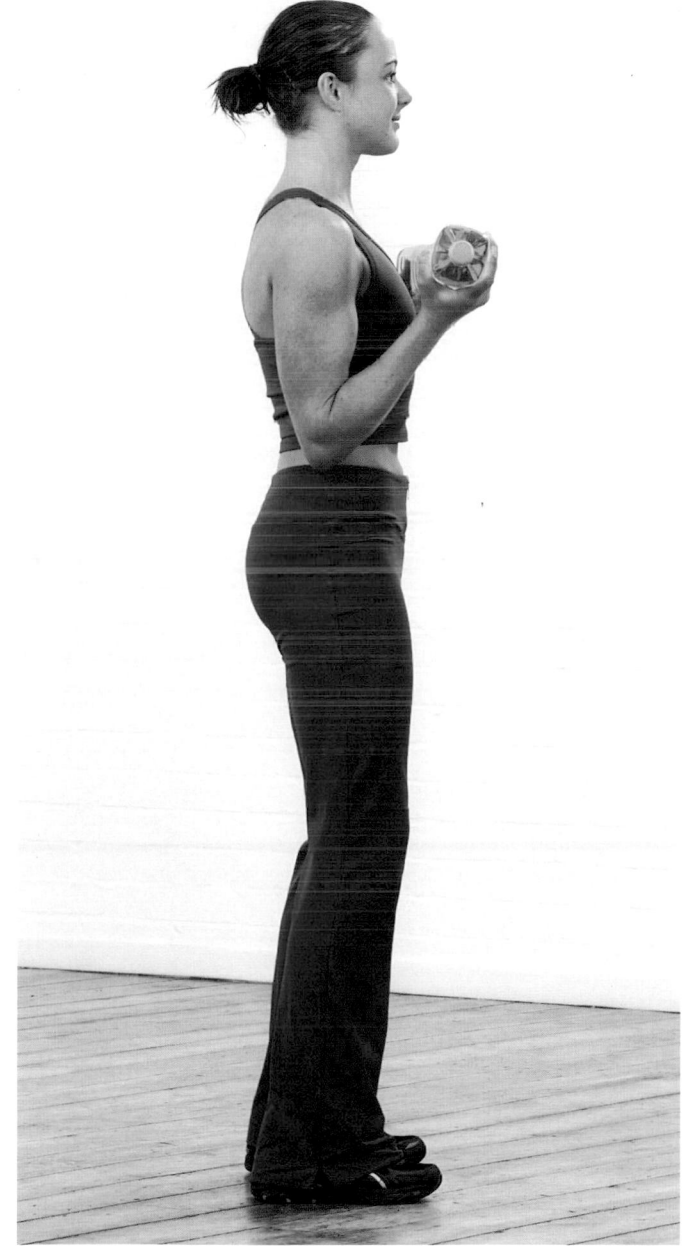

2   Slowly lower the weights back down to the starting position. For such a simple exercise, it is amazing how many people get it wrong.

Arms—Beginners

bench dips

Area Worked: Back of the arms and front of the shoulders.
Name of Muscles: Triceps and Anterior Deltoid.

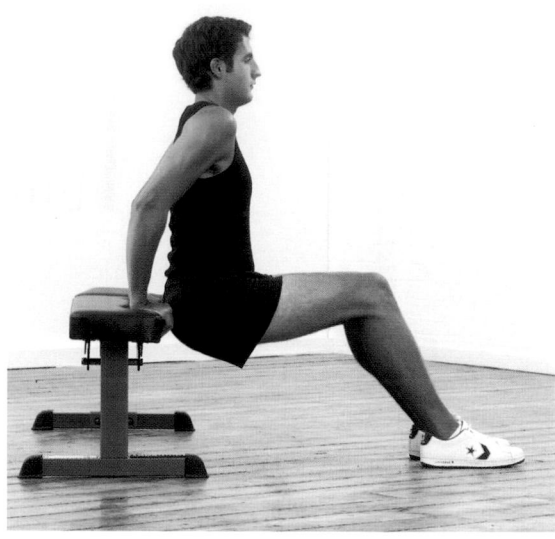
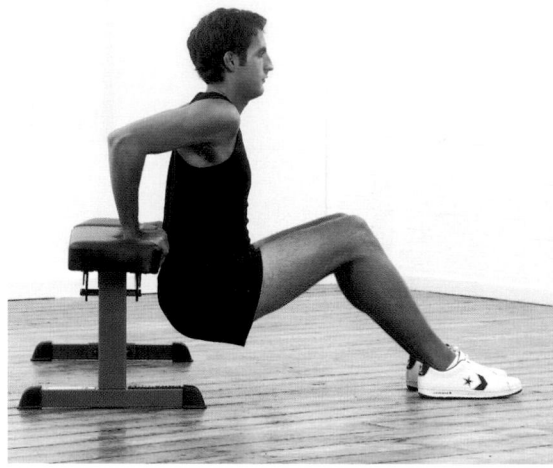

1 Sit on the edge of your chosen object—e.g. a bench, a chair—with your palms gripping the edge by your thighs.

2 Take the weight on your hands and move your upper body just clear of the edge. Bend the elbows and lower yourself toward the floor.

Hints & Tips

- You can use pretty much any type of chair or seat you have at hand, so long as it is not too high or too low. If you sit in it you should have somewhere around a 90-degree bend in your knee. If you have that, you have your dipping station. Obviously, do not use a chair with wheels!

- To make the exercise harder, move your feet farther away from you; but make sure that you keep your hips pushed back and your back stays straight.

Technique

- Keep your weight over the arms by pushing your butt and hips back toward the equipment you are using.

- Try to keep the back straight as you lower yourself and when pushing back up.

- Keep the elbows soft at the top of the movement and keep it smooth.

- Keep a 90-degree bend at the knees and keep the feet flat to start with. This can be changed as your strength increases.

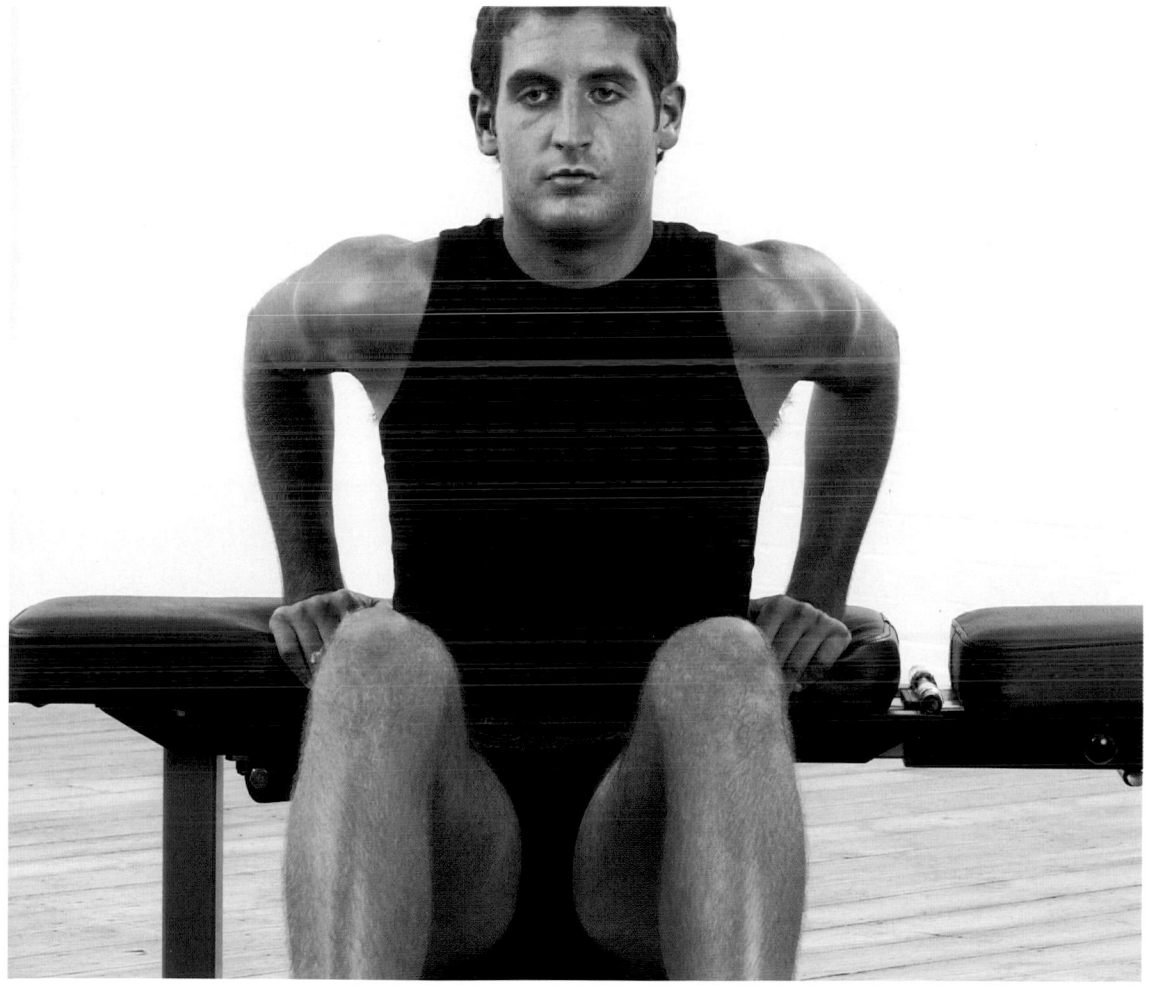

3 Push with your hands to lift you back up.

Arms—Beginners

supinated tricep extension

Area Worked: Back of the arms.
Name of Muscle: Tricep.

1 With a weight in each hand, lie on the floor on your back. Your knees should be bent and your feet flat.

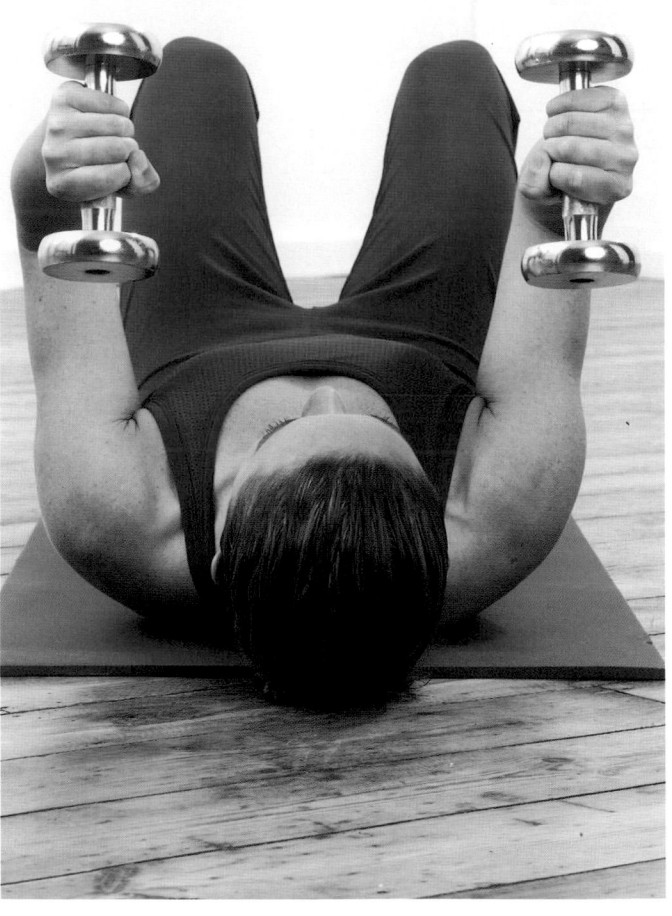

Hints & Tips

- Don't drop the weights! This should be at the top of your "things not to do" list. So if you are perspiring a little, it may be an idea to give your palms a wipe.

- Keep it slow as you lower the weight. The lower you go, the heavier the weight will feel, so be prepared for this.

- The weight should be at shoulder-width, not over your face. (See hint number one, above.)

Technique

- When lying on the floor try not to relax. You are keeping the body tight to stabilize you during the exercise.

- Your upper arms should stay vertical through the exercise. Try not to move them forward or back.

- At the lowest point of the exercise you should have about a 90-degree bend at the elbow. When you straighten the arm, be careful not to lock the elbow joints. As so often with upper body exercises, keep them soft.

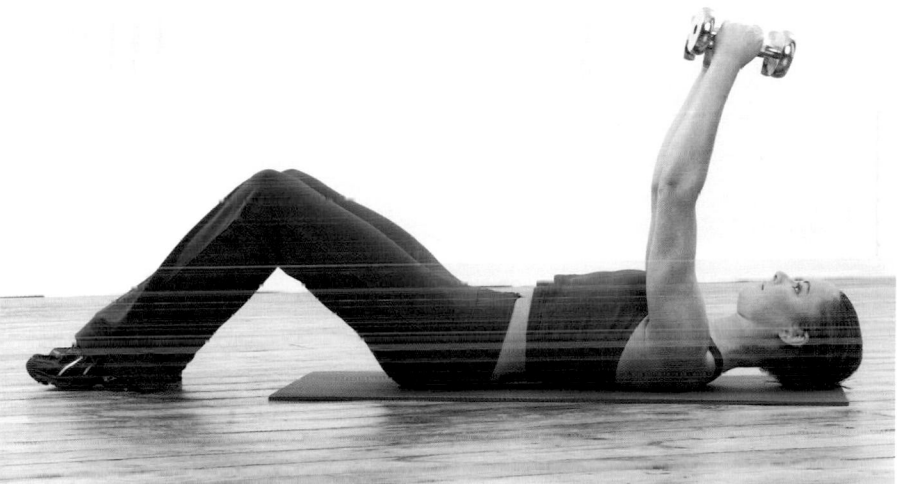

2 Put your arms straight up over your chest. Keeping the elbows where they are, lower the weights down toward your shoulders.

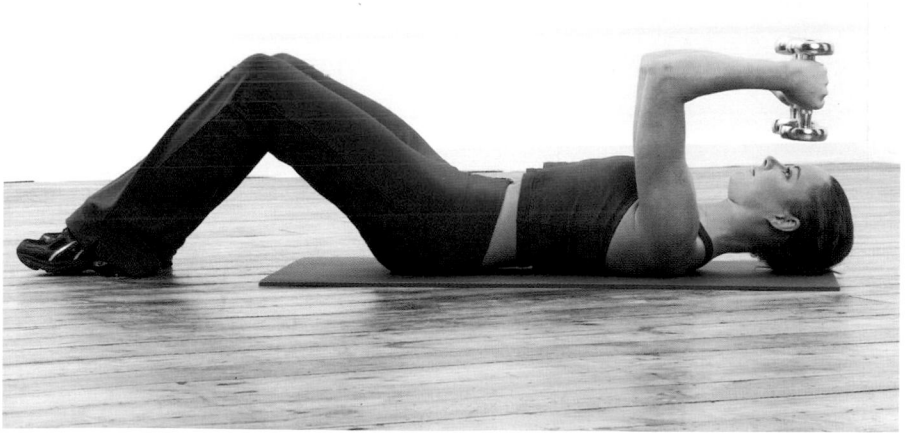

3 Pause for a second and then straighten the arms again.

Arms—Advanced

zottman curl

Area Worked: Front of arms and forearms.
Name of Muscles: Biceps and Wrist Extensors.

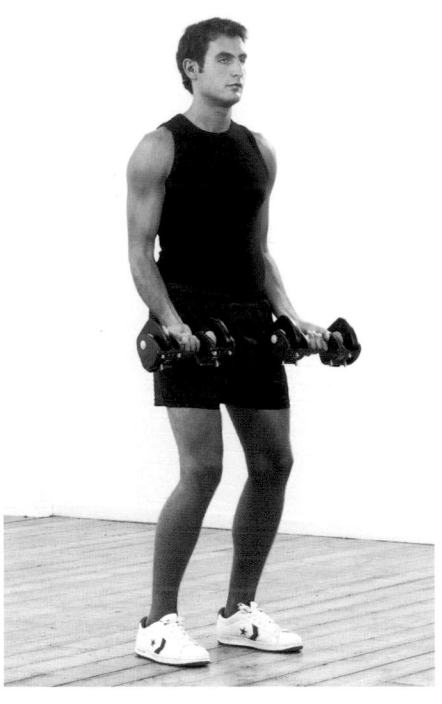 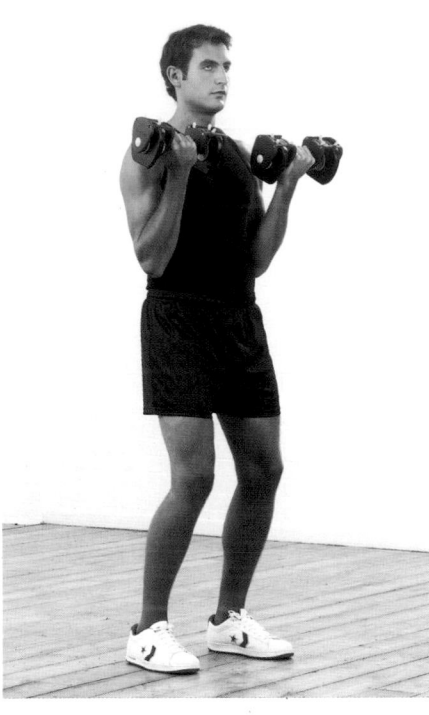

1 Stand tall, holding the weights by your sides with the palms facing forward.

2 Bend the elbows and curl the weights up toward your shoulders.

Hints & Tips

• There is a lot more technique to this exercise than the standard Bicep Curl, so practice with a lighter weight to get the technique and then start to add the weight when you feel confident.

• You can do both arms at the same time, or do them alternately to really concentrate on each arm individually.

Technique

- Fix the elbows at your sides. Do not let them move out or forward during the exercise.

- Complete the rotation of the wrist just before you reach the top of the movement and really focus on the squeeze. |

You should feel the muscle get tighter as you lift.

- Fix the wrists. Do not let them drop back when you lift, or forward when you lower down.

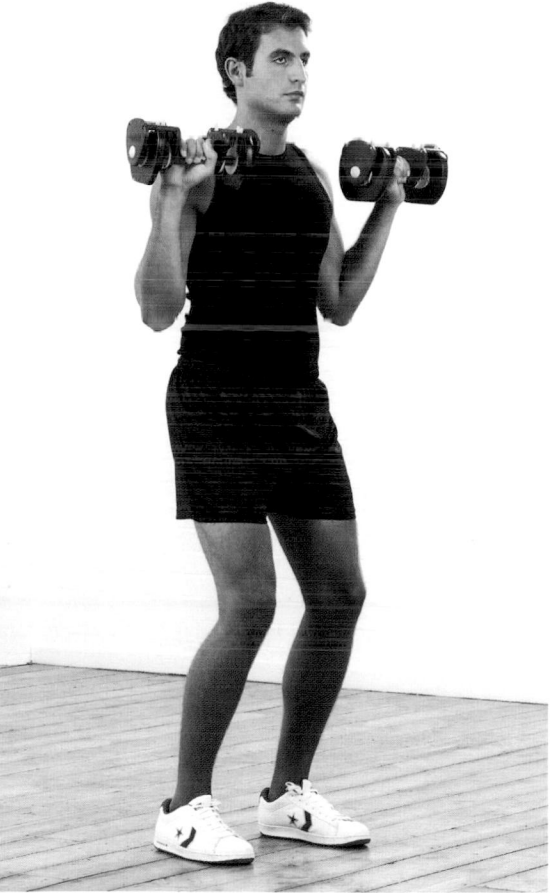

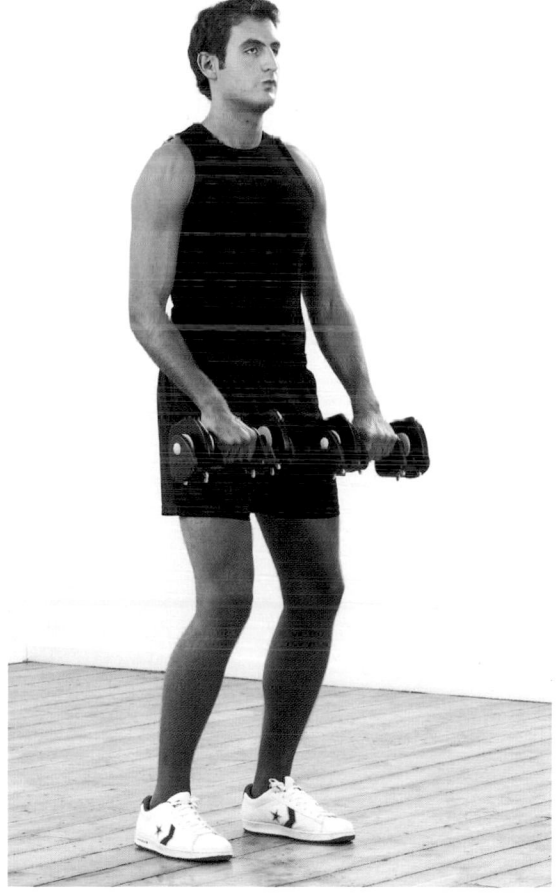

3 Rotate the wrist so that the palm is facing down and lower the weights back to your sides, knuckles facing forward.

4 Rotate the wrist so that the palms face forward and repeat.

Arms—Advanced

raised dip

Area Worked: Back of the arm and front of the shoulder.
Name of Muscles: Triceps and Anterior Deltoid.

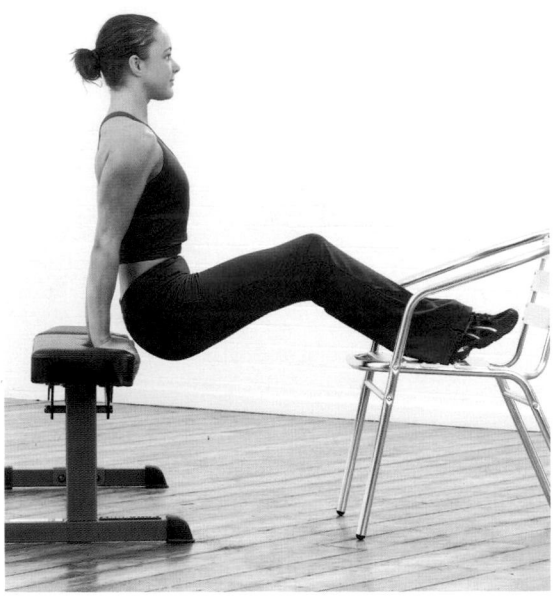

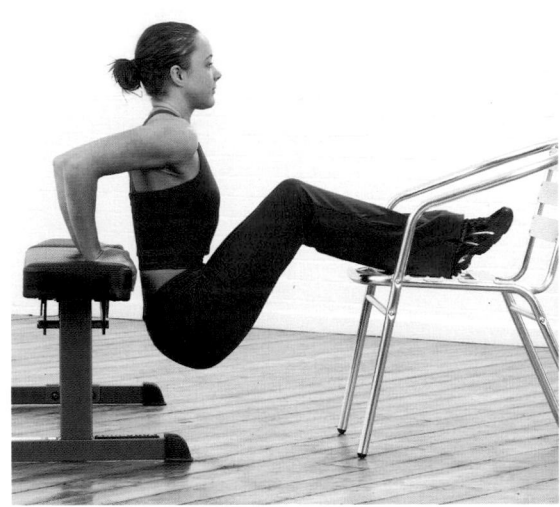

1 Sit on the edge of your chosen object (step, chair, or bench) with your palms gripping the edge by your thighs. Place your feet on a stable object of similar height.

2 Bend the elbows and lower yourself toward the floor.

Hints & Tips

- If you would really like a challenge, try putting both your feet on top of a ball or even a ball for each foot. This will destabilize you and make the muscles work harder to fix you in place. It doesn't matter about the size—soccer balls or basketballs would be about right, and a tennis ball would not destabilize or raise the feet enough.

Technique

- Raising your feet makes it harder as your center of gravity is now higher. If you feel uncertain, start by raising them a little, as even that can make a substantial difference to the difficulty.

- Keep your weight over the arms by pushing your butt and hips back toward the equipment you are using.

- Try to keep the back straight as you lower yourself down and when you are pushing back up.

- Keep the elbows soft at the top of the movement and keep it smooth.

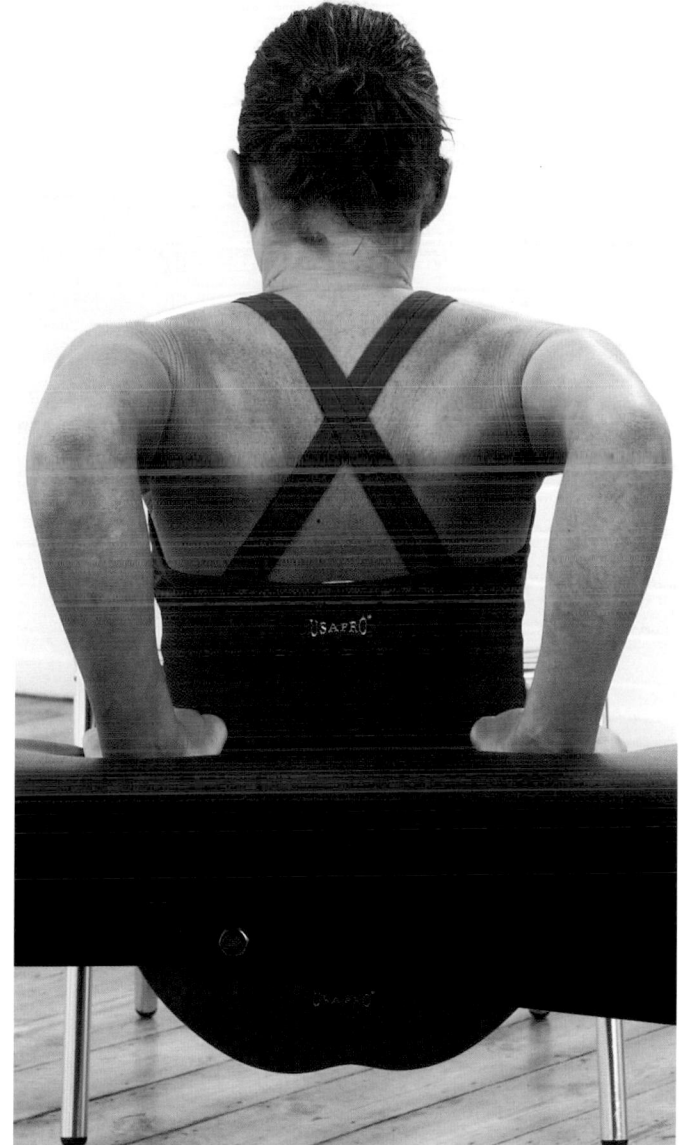

3 Push with your hands to lift you back up.

Arms—Advanced

knuckled close grip press up

Area Worked: Back of the arms, chest, and shoulders. (Abdominals stabilizing).
Name of Muscles: Triceps, Pectorals, and Anterior Deltoid.

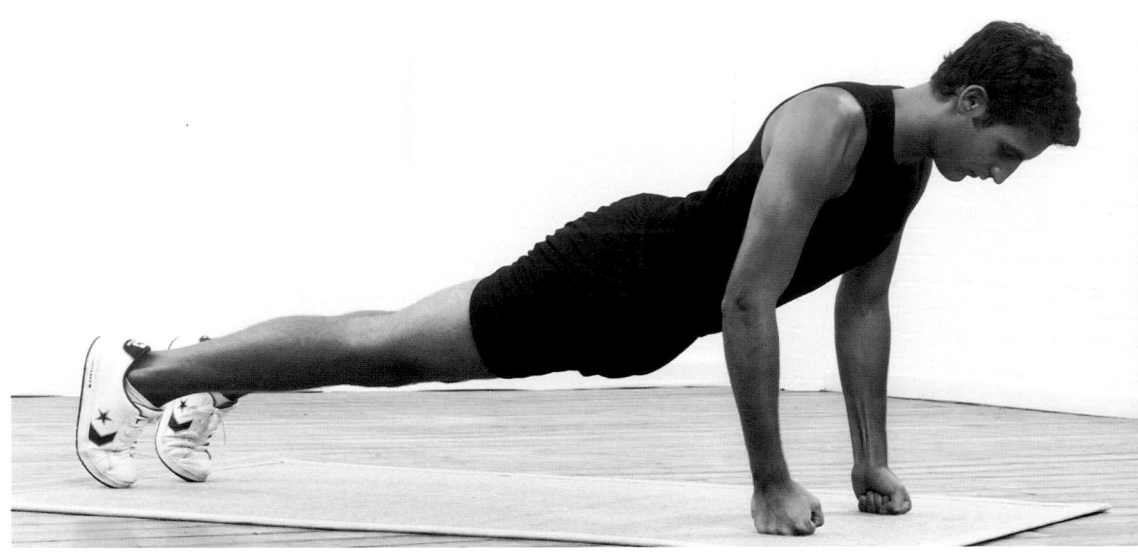

1 Place yourself on the floor on your hands and knees. Position your hands at approximately shoulder width and close your hands so that you are now supporting yourself on your knuckles. Your palms should be facing inward. Walk the knees back.

Hints & Tips

• Lower your whole body on each repetition, not just your chest. Your body should be in one straight line from head to toes.

• Try not to push your head forward. Your gauge is how low your chest goes, not how far forward you can push your head. If you feel uncertain, find someone who can check your position, as it can sometimes be hard to tell when you are performing the exercise.

Technique

- Keep the wrists fixed. By moving on to your knuckles you have a smaller contact point with the floor, making the exercise harder and also making you less stable.

- The body should be in a straight line from shoulders to feet. Try not to push your butt in the air and keep the abdominal muscles braced tight to stop your hips from dropping.

- Keep the elbows tucked into your ribs as you lower and lift. As you become fatigued, they will try to flare out to recruit more from the chest muscles. Keep them in tight to really work the back of the arms.

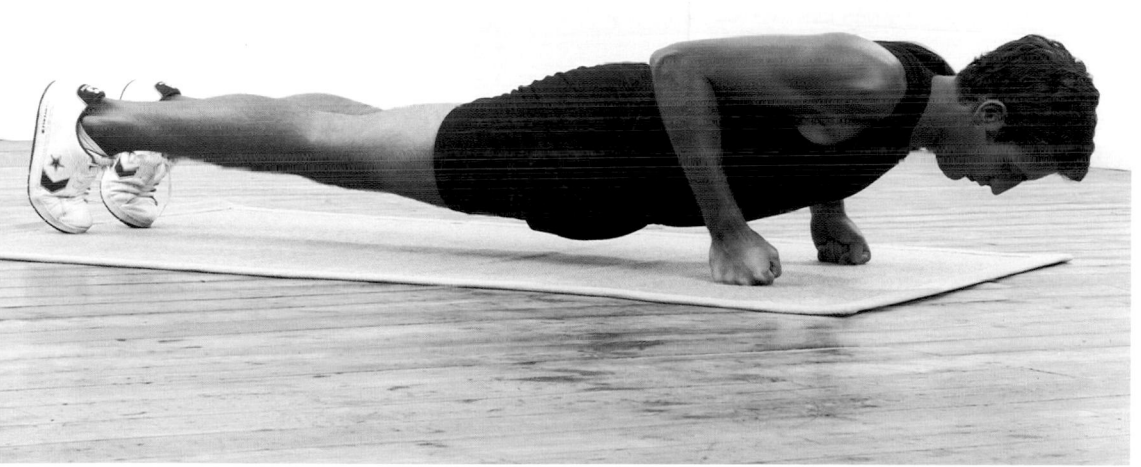

2 When you are supported by your toes and fists, bend the elbow and lower your chest down toward the floor. Push to straighten the arms to lift yourself back up to the starting position.

Shoulders—Beginners

shoulder press

Area Worked: Shoulders and back of the arms.
Name of Muscles: Deltoid and Triceps.

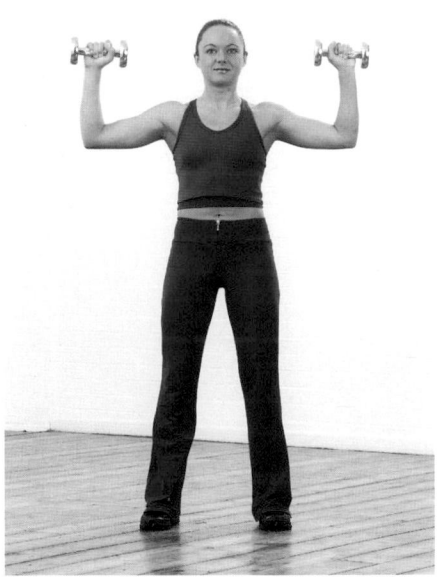 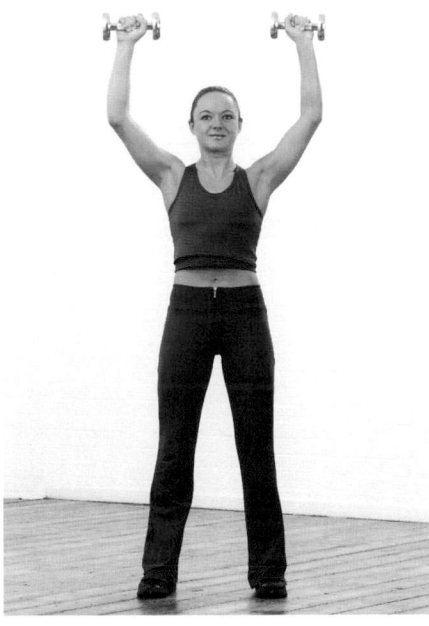

1 Hold a weight in each hand and lift them up so that they are level with your eyes and your palms are facing forward.

2 Push the weights up over your head until your arms are almost straight and the weights almost touch.

Hints & Tips

- This is an exercise that can be done either sitting or standing. Whichever you choose, remember your posture. Stay tall and don't let your back round; and if you are standing, mind the ceiling!

- The shoulder muscles tend not to give you very much warning when they are about to fatigue, so be careful with the weight. The weight that seems easy for the first half of your set may suddenly become a whole lot more challenging in the second half.

Technique

- Try to keep the elbows back, in line with your upper body.

- The forearms should stay vertical throughout the movement. Be careful the weights do not pull you to the sides, forward, or back. They should feel balanced.

- When pushing, do not lock the elbows. Keep them soft at the top.

- When you lower the weight back to about eye level you should have around a 90-degree bend at your elbows. If not, adjust the height as necessary, but do not come too low as this may but excessive strain on the shoulder joint.

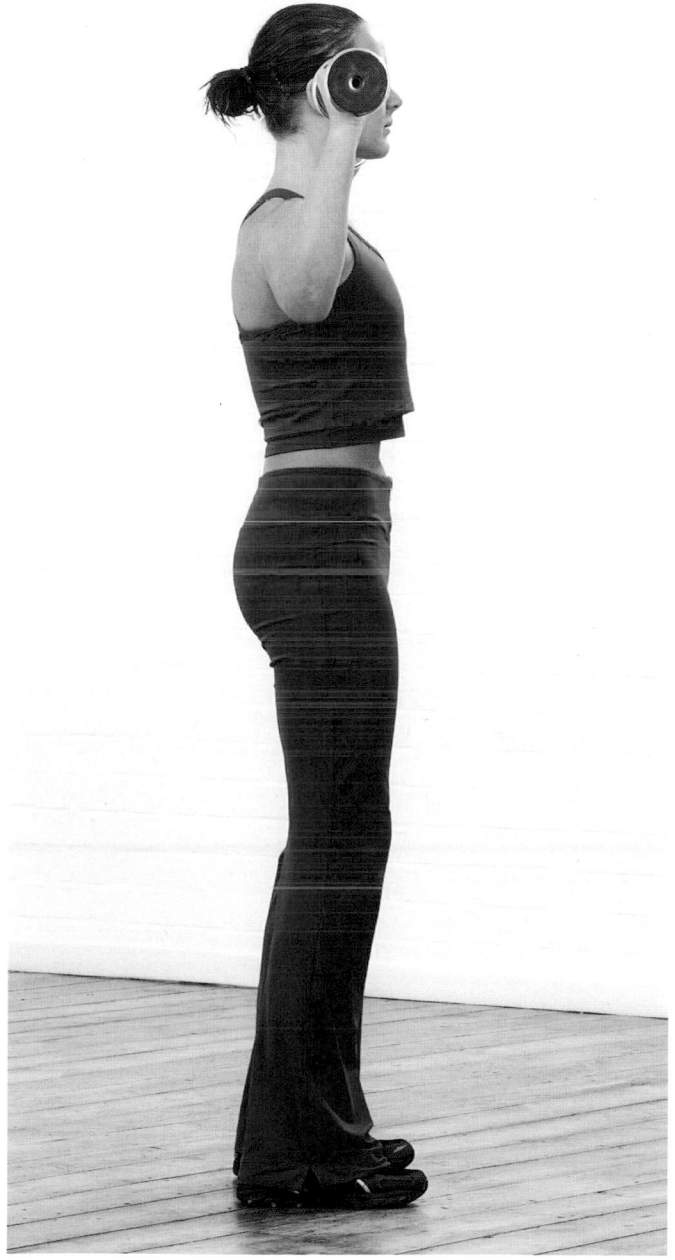

3 Slowly lower the weights back down until they are back at eye level.

Shoulders–Beginners

lateral raise

Area Worked: Shoulders.
Name of Muscle: Medial Deltoid.

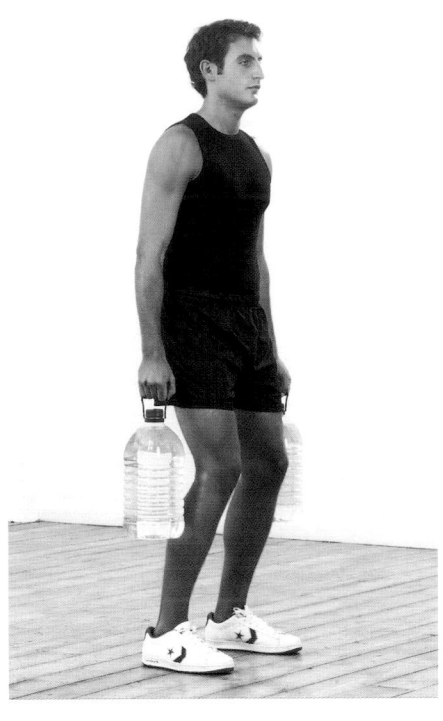 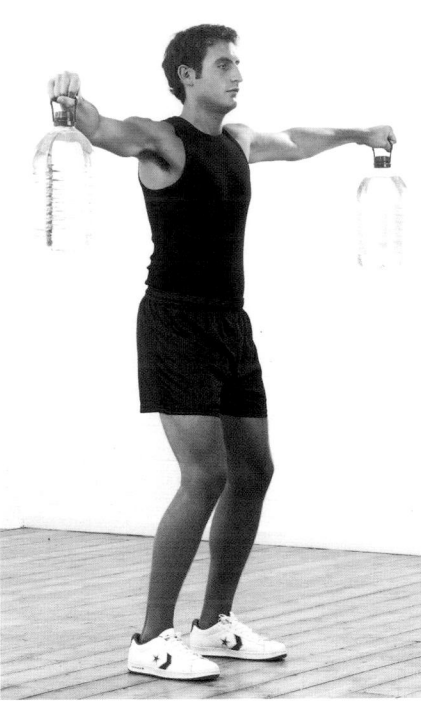

1 Hold a weight in each hand, palms inward, so that they are almost resting on your thighs. Place a slight bend in your elbows.

2 Lift the weights out to the side in a smooth arc until your elbows and the weights are level with your shoulders.

Hints & Tips

- As you lift the weight rotate your wrist slightly inward as if you were pouring water from a glass. This will emphasize the medial head of your deltoids.

- Again, this is an exercise that can be done either sitting or standing. Whichever you choose, remember your posture and stay tall.

Technique

- Fix the bend in your elbow. It should neither increase nor decrease throughout the exercise.

- Keep the elbows pointing behind you throughout the movement. As the exercise becomes harder your elbows will want to point to the floor. This will take the emphasis off the muscle that you are trying to work.

- Keep the wrists fixed straight. Do not let them flop.

- Do not let the weights rest at the bottom of the movement. Keep a gap between your legs and the weights at the bottom of the movement.

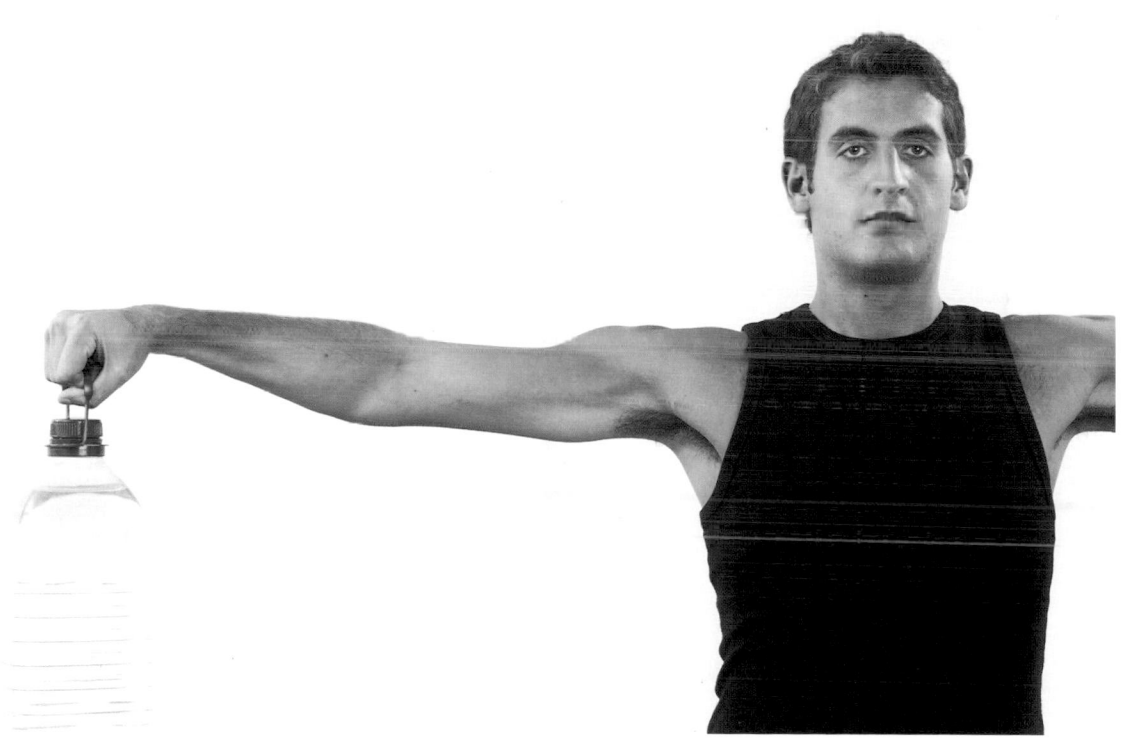

3 Slowly lower the weights back through the same range of movement.

Shoulders—Beginners

front raise

Area Worked: Shoulders.
Name of Muscle: Anterior Deltoid.

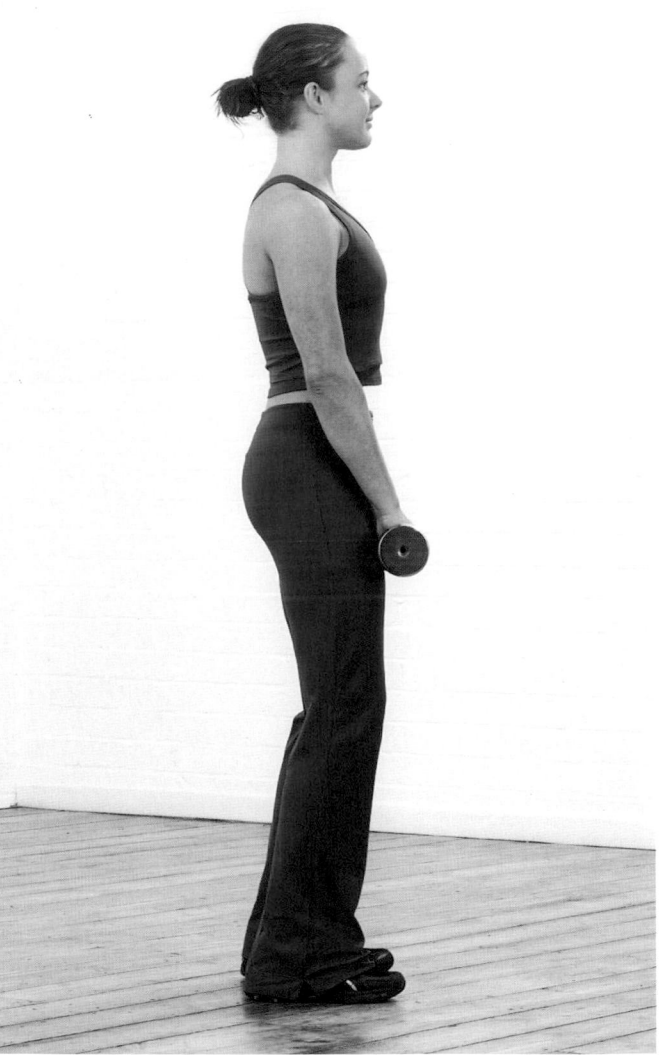

1 Hold the weights in front of your thighs, with your palms facing your thighs.

Hints & Tips

- This exercise can be done by lifting both arms together or lifting alternately. Lifting together does put more pressure on your lower back so if you feel uncertain, try alternating or starting very light.

- As your shoulders start to fatigue you will feel yourself starting to arch your back to lift the weights. To avoid this, consciously tighten the abdominals and soften the knees. If this still doesn't help, then your shoulders have done as much as they can.

Technique

- Keep the hands and weights at shoulder-width throughout the exercise.

- Keep a slight bend in the elbows and fix the wrists so that they are straight.

- Keep the knees soft and the abdominals tight.

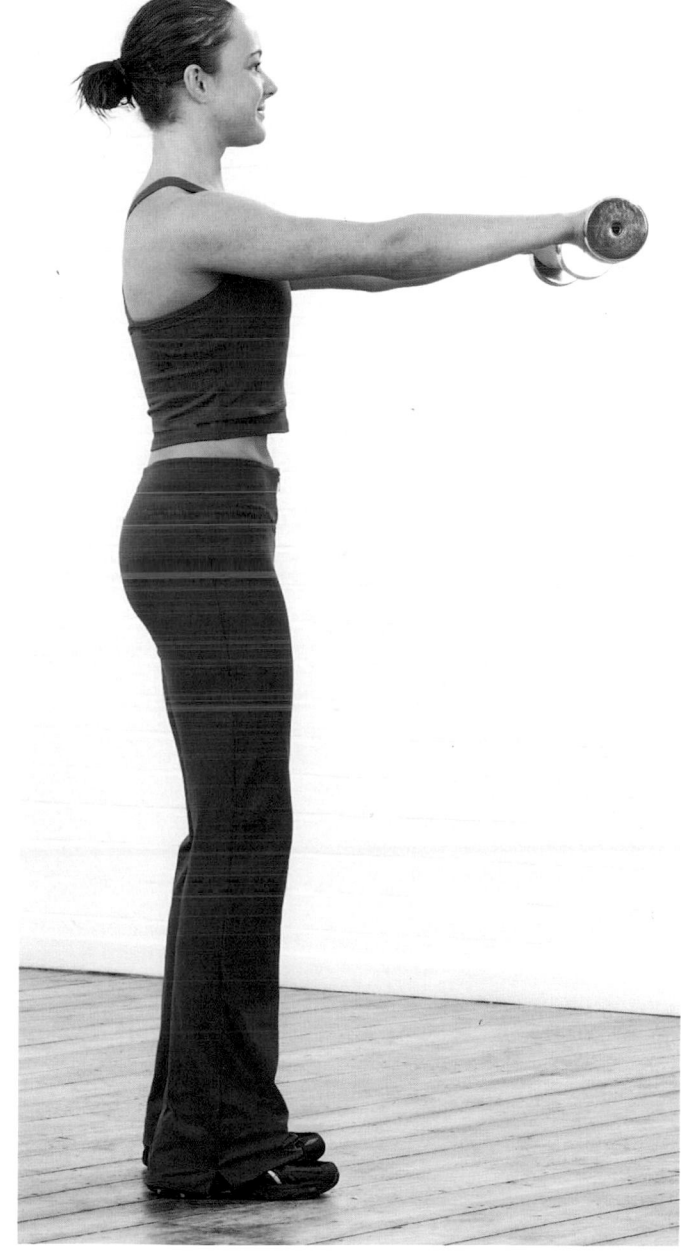

2 Lift the weight out in front through a smooth arc to shoulder height. Slowly lower the weights back down in front of your thighs.

Shoulders—Advanced

corkscrew shoulder press

Area Worked: Shoulders and back of arms.
Name of Muscles: Deltoids and Triceps.

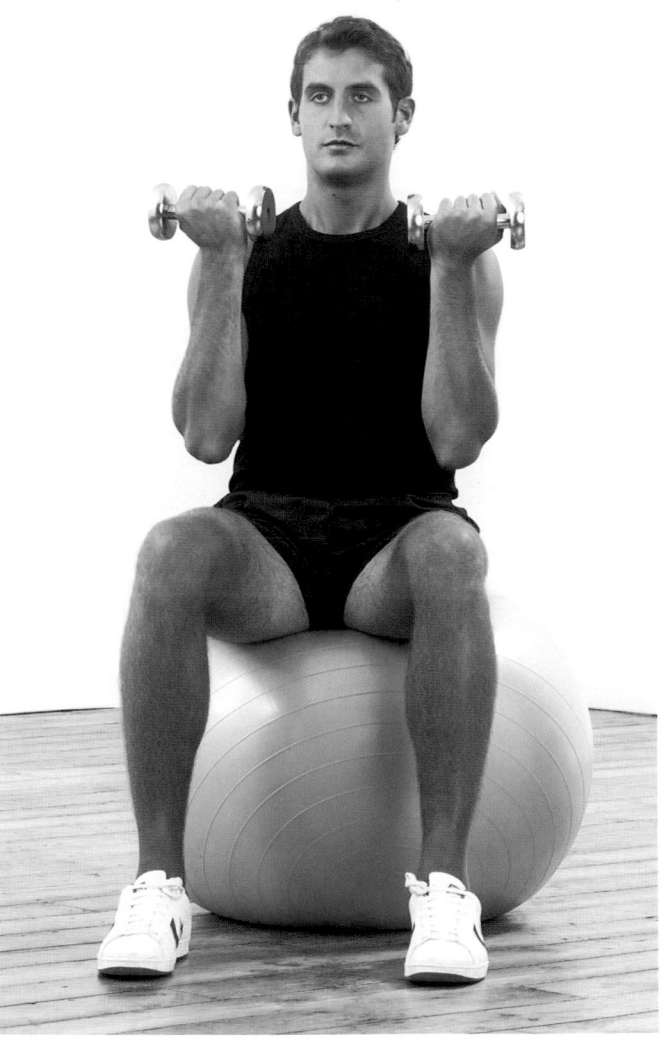

1 Hold a weight in each hand in front of you at shoulder height. Your elbows should be tucked in near your ribs with your palms facing you.

Hints & Tips

- Like the earlier Shoulder Press, this can be done either sitting or standing. Whichever you choose, remember your posture. Stay tall, do not let your back round. Think of the exercises as three separate phases you are combining. The first phase is pushing up with palms facing. The second is rotating your elbows back and the third is a final push with elbows back and your palms forward.

- Keep the movement constant and smooth by always pushing the weights up during the three phases.

Technique

- Try to keep the exercise as one smooth movement when pushing and lowering the weight.

- When you are at the bottom of the movement with your elbows near your ribs try not to rest your elbows against your body. This will keep the shoulders working throughout the exercise.

- Be careful not to lock your elbows when straightening the arms. Keep the joint soft.

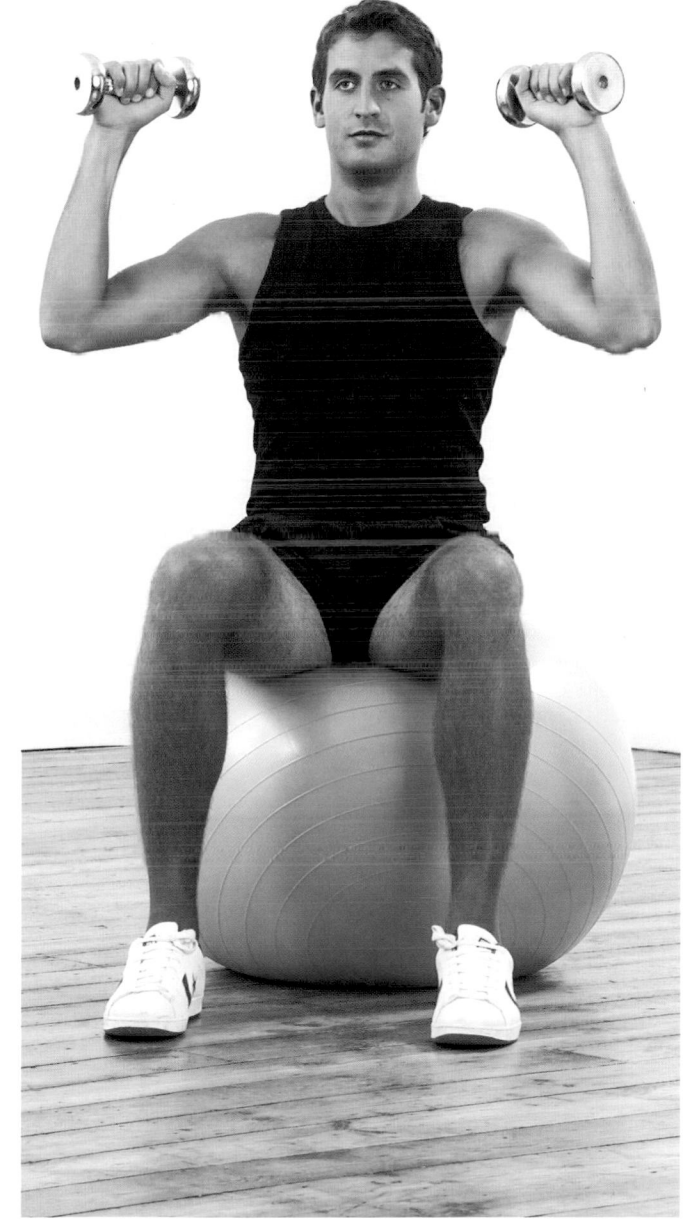

2 Push the weights up and rotate the hands and elbows out and back so the weights are now at your sides.

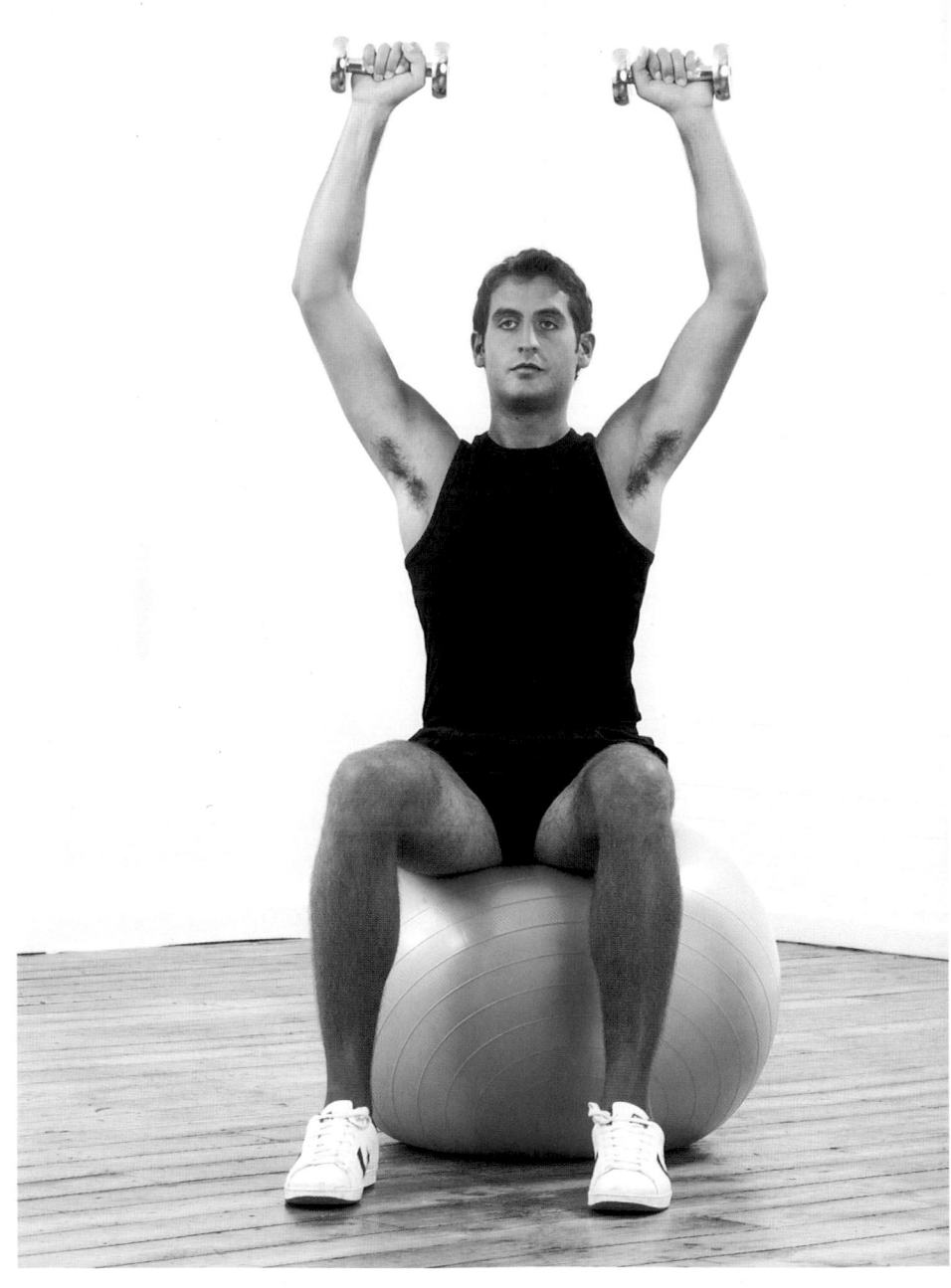

3 Left Continue pushing up until the dumbbells almost touch above your head.

4 and 5 Lower the weights back down in the same range of movement. As you lower the weights, take them out to the sides and then rotate the hands and elbows in again near the ribs.

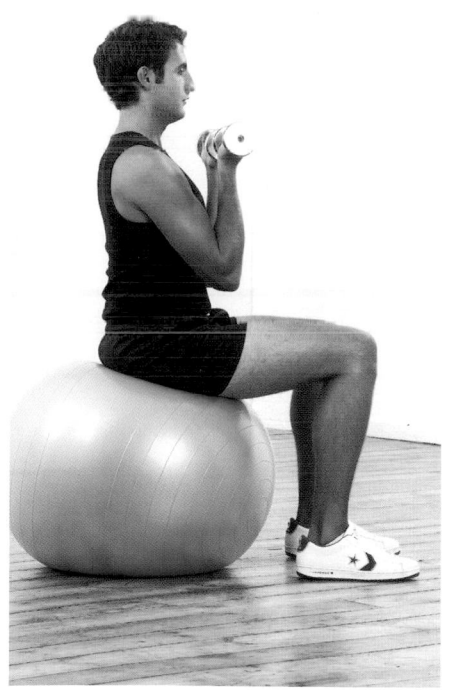

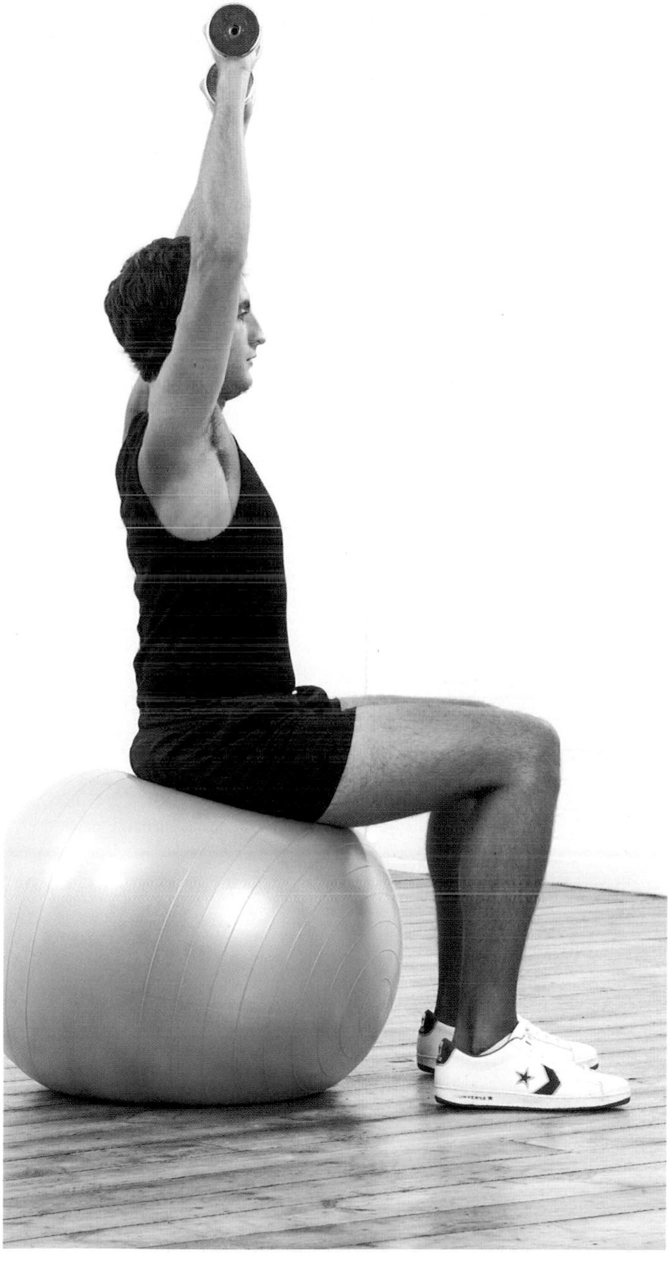

Shoulders—Advanced

upright row

Area Worked: Shoulders, upper back, and the front of the arms.
Name of Muscles: Deltoids, Trapezius, and Biceps.

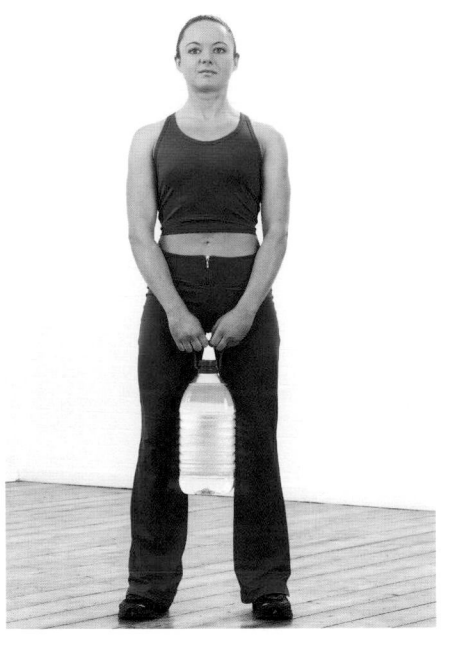
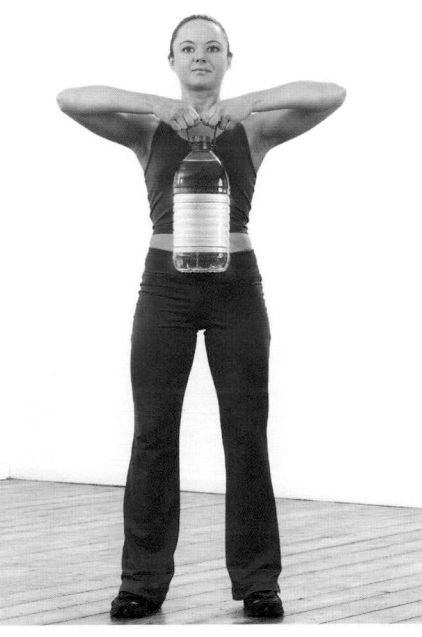

1 Stand tall, holding the weights in front of your thighs with your palms facing you.

2 Leading with the elbows, pull the weights up the front of your body until the weights are approximately level with your chest and your elbows are at shoulder height.

Hints & Tips

• There is nothing to be gained by lifting your elbows any higher than your shoulders and it will in fact make the exercise slightly easier. Focus on your range of movement. Keep it smooth and consistent for each repetition.

• As your muscles start to fatigue it will become tempting to use your lower back as leverage to lift the weight. If this happens it simply means your shoulders have done as much as they can; so put the weights down and move on to the next exercise.

Technique

- Keep the knees soft and brace the body. Because the weights are in front of you this means that your body is going to feel like it is being pulled forward. This is opposed by the muscles in your lower back, so keep your mid-section braced.

- When the weights are at the bottom keep a slight bend in the elbows to keep the muscles under tension.

- Keep the wrists relaxed and focus on pulling with your elbows. The elbows should always be above your wrists during the lifting and lowering phases.

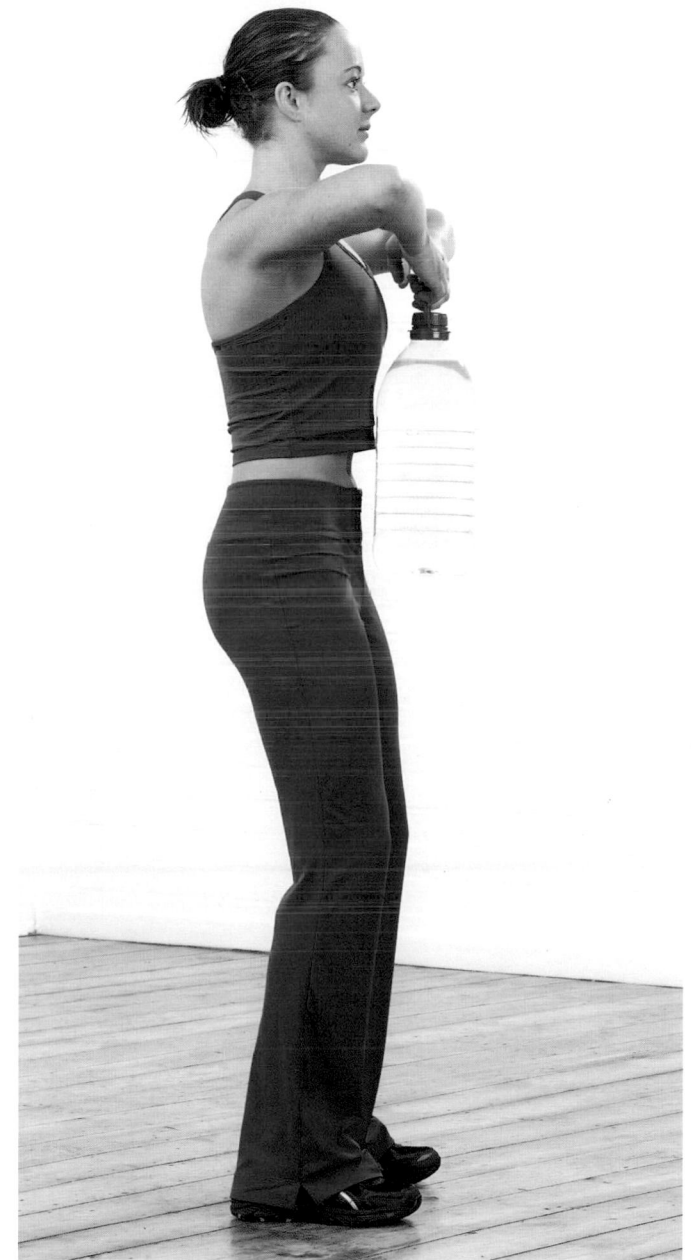

3 Slowly lower the weights back down to the start position.

Shoulders—Advanced

round the world

Area Worked: Shoulders.
Name of Muscles: Deltoids.

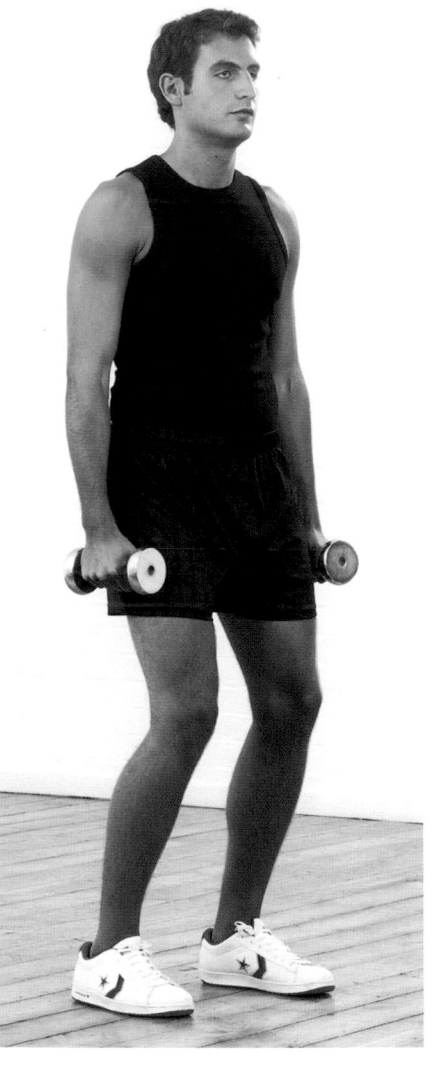

1 Stand tall and hold a weight in each hand.

2 Keeping a slight bend in the elbow, raise the weights out to the side up to shoulder height.

Hints & Tips

- This is essentially a combination of the Lateral and the Front Raise exercises. But because you are keeping the arms at shoulder height in the middle of the movement, your muscles are under tension for much longer, so bear this in mind when selecting the weight you are going to use. Start light!

Technique

- Keep the wrists fixed and the elbows soft throughout the movement.

- Keep the body fixed and the knees soft. Do not arch the back and keep those abdominal muscles braced.

- Keep looking straight ahead. Avoid the temptation to look down when it starts to get tough!

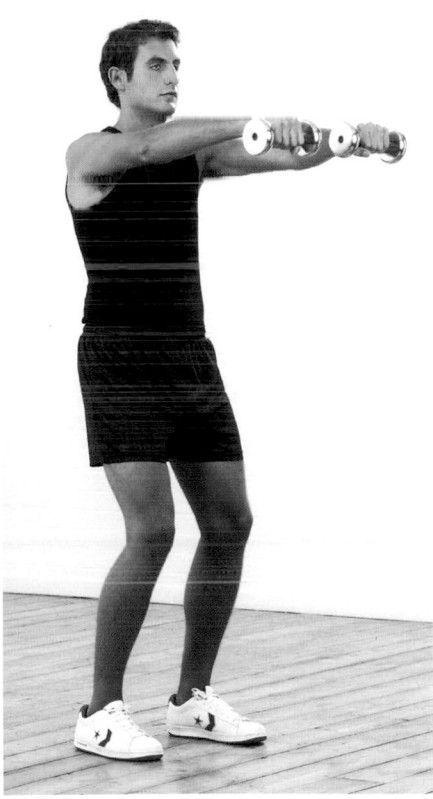

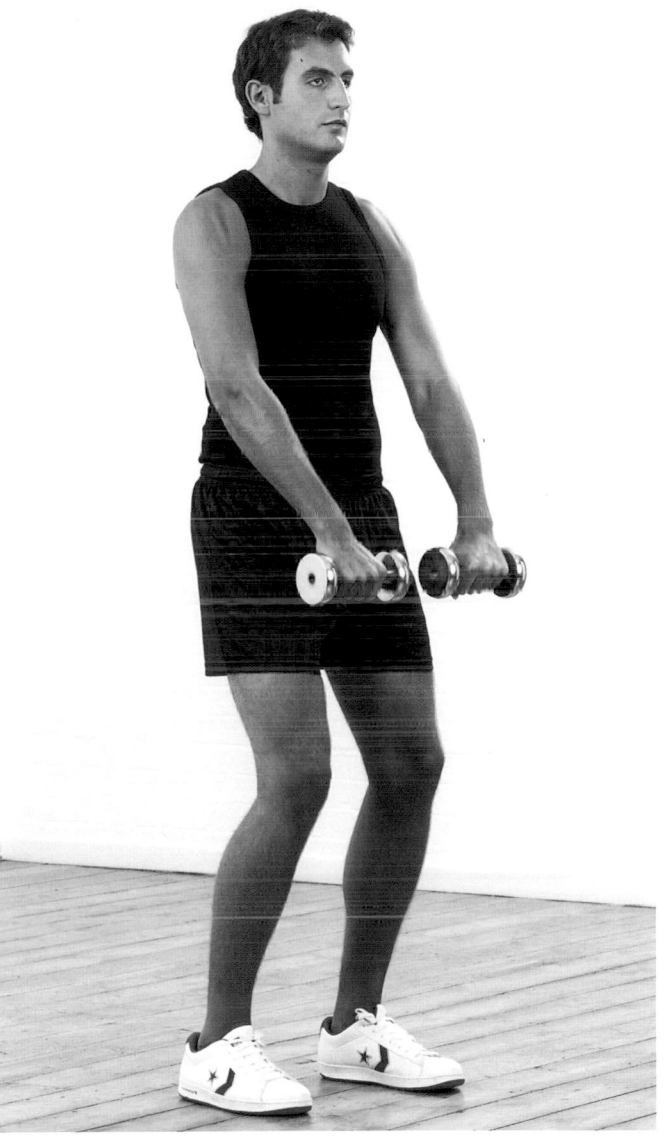

3 Maintaining the weights at shoulder height move the arms around to the front of your body so that your hands are at about shoulder width. Lower the weight back down toward your thighs and leave a slight gap. Your palms now face the front of your thighs.

4 To complete the repetition, reverse the movement so that you lift up from the front to shoulder height. Take the arms back round to your sides and lower the weights.

Abs/Back—Beginners

half bridge

Area Worked: Stomach.
Name of Muscles: Transverse Abdominus and Rectus Abdominus.

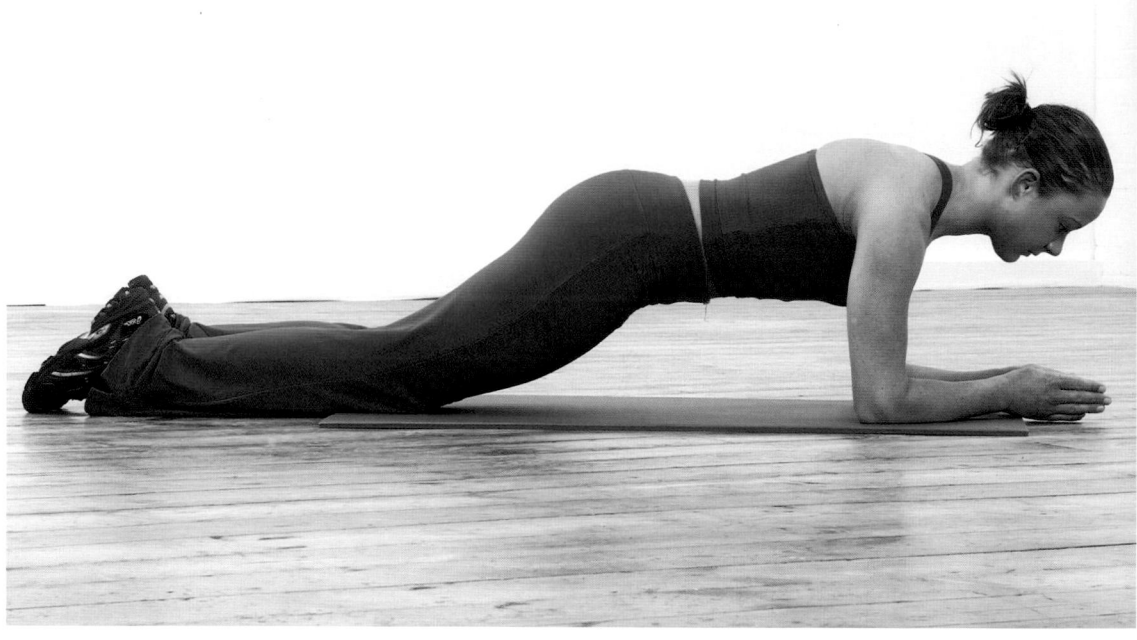

1 Position yourself on the floor, face down, supporting your weight on your forearms and your knees. Walk the knees back until you have as near a straight line as you can get through your shoulders, hips, and knees. Hold this position.

Hints & Tips

• Hold the position for as long as you can. There will come a point where your muscles will fatigue and this is usually a gradual process. As your abdominal muscles fatigue you will start to feel discomfort in your lower back. Stop the exercise when you feel this happen. Do not be tempted to carry on: your abdominal muscles have done as much as they can.

Technique

- Keep your elbows below your shoulders and make your hands into fists, bringing them together to make a triangle. You should feel stable in this position.

- Keep the knees apart the width of your hips during the exercise.

- Be careful not to let your hips drop towards the floor. Keep your abdominal muscles pulled in tight.

- Don't push your butt in the air. You should have a straight line from shoulders to knees.

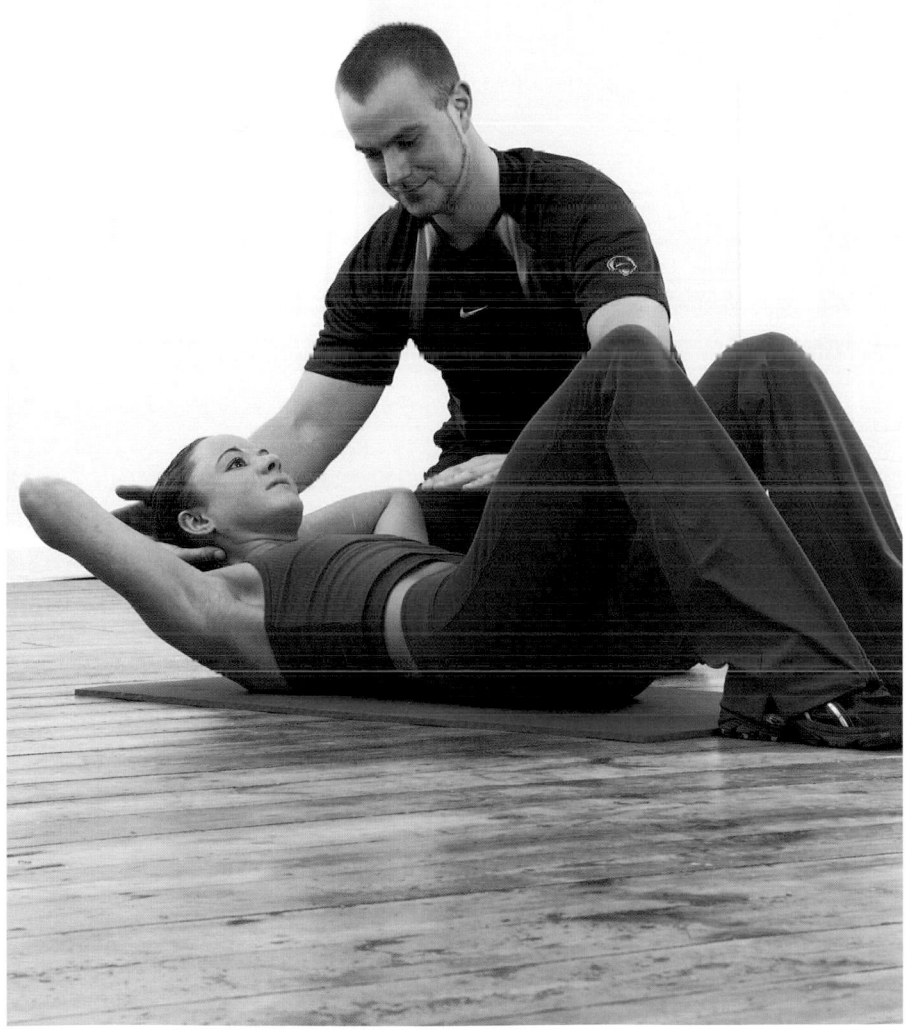

What do we want? Flat abs! When do we want 'em? Now! A general point: perhaps the most desired body change is also the one that is helped most by "on-the-spot" input from a partner. It is so easy either to "cheat" when performing abdominal exercises, or simply to do them ineffectively.

Abs/Back–Beginners

abdominal curl

Area Worked: Front of stomach (upper).
Name of Muscle: Rectus Abdominus.

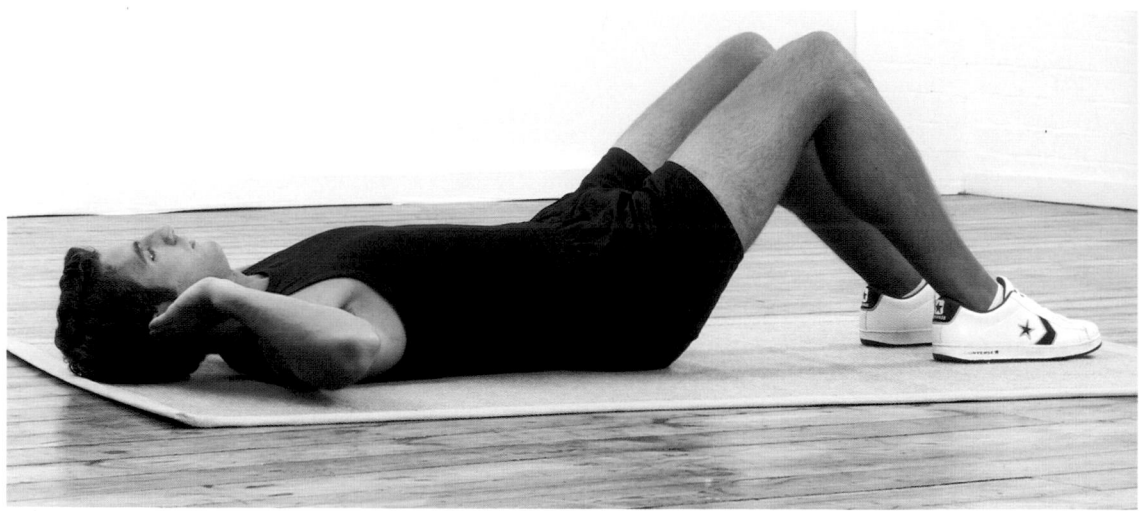

1 Lie on your back with your knees bent and your feet flat on the floor. Curl up, lifting your shoulder blades off the floor while keeping your lower back and feet in contact with the floor.

Hints & Tips

- Hand position has a huge impact on how difficult the exercise is. The following list runs from easiest to hardest. hands on thighs—hands across the chest—fingertips at temples (elbows forward)—fingertips at temples (elbows back)—hands over head.

- To check you are pulling the muscles in when you lift, place one hand on your abdomen and gently push with your fingertips. Do a couple of repetitions with your stomach pulled in and make a mental note of how it feels. Now do a couple of repetitions and consciously push your muscles out. Make sure you know how each one feels. When doing the exercise occasionally check using this technique to make sure that the muscles are always being pulled in.

Technique

- Pull your abdominal muscles in as you curl up.

- Keep a small gap, approximately the size of your fist, between your chin and your chest and try not to push your head forward as you curl up.

- You only need to lift a few inches from the floor. Do not feel the need to try to go higher.

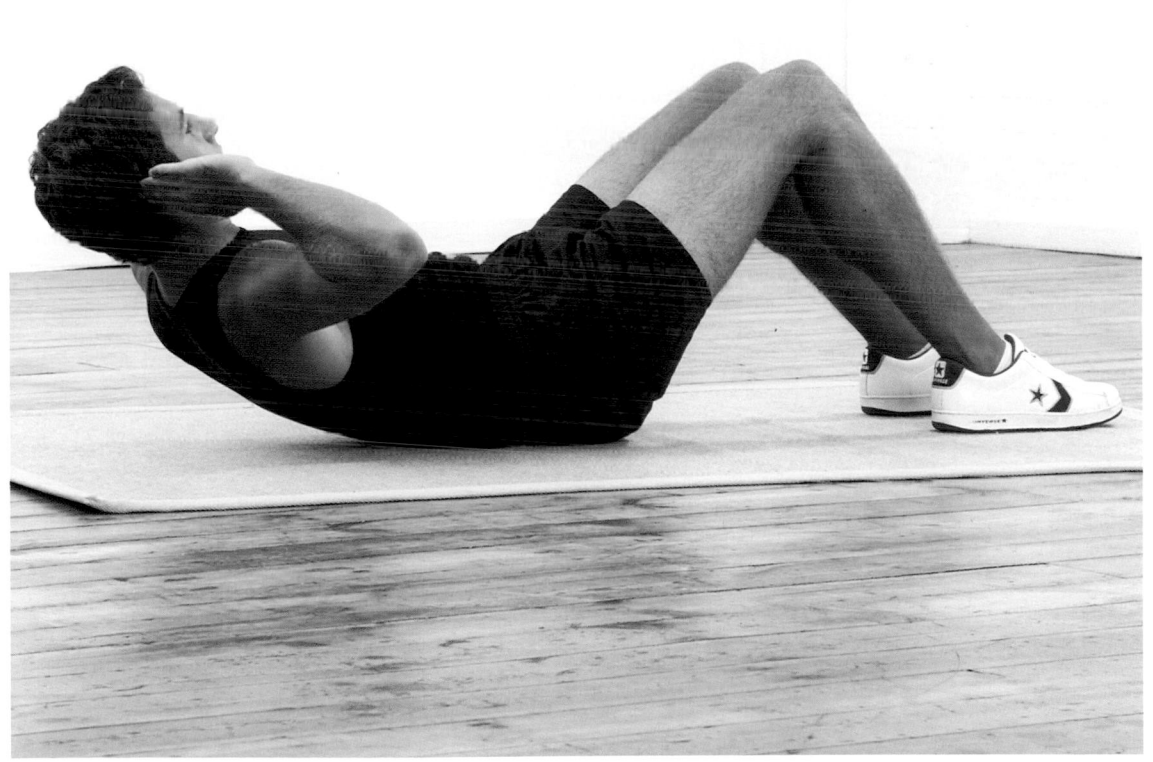

2 Slowly lower back down, leaving a small gap between the floor and your upper back, then repeat the movement.

Abs/Back—Beginners

oblique curl

Area Worked: Sides of stomach (waist).
Name of Muscles: Obliques.

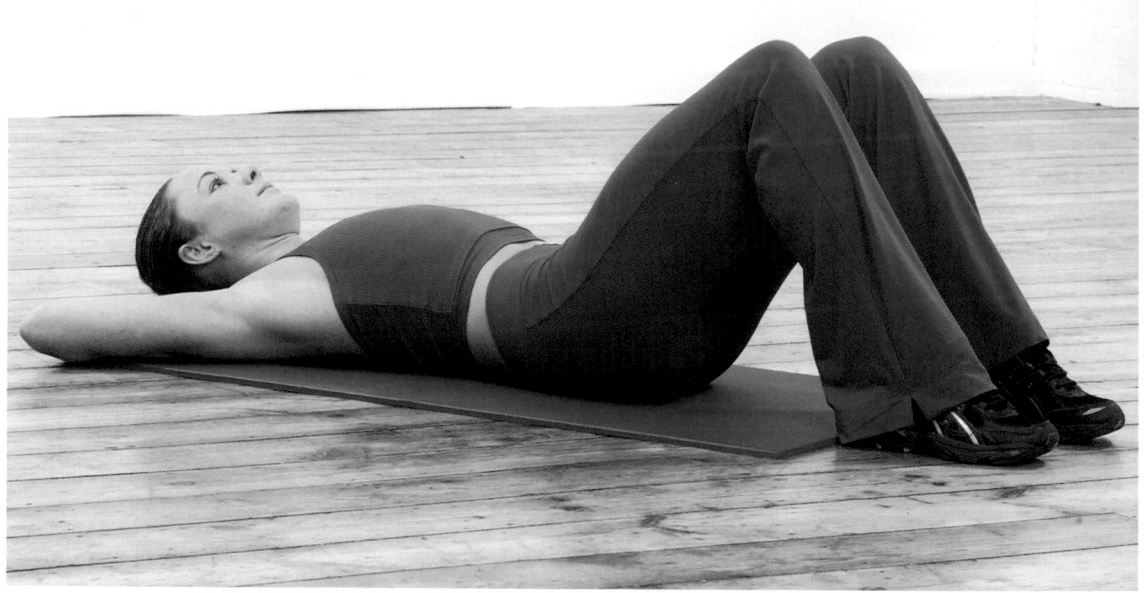

1 Lie on your back with your knees bent and your feet flat on the floor.

Hints & Tips

• Do not throw yourself up into the movement. In just about every exercise, you are trying to make the muscle work as hard as it can and to do this you must retain full control of the movement. If you launch yourself quickly you generate momentum. The more momentum you generate, the less work your muscles have to do; and ultimately, the less benefit you will get.

Technique

- Pull your abdominal muscles in as you curl up.

- Keep a small gap, approximately the size of your fist, between your chin and your chest and try not to push your head forward as you curl up. This can put a bad strain on the neck.

- Keep the movement as one smooth lift. Start the initial lift straight and then slowly rotate the upper body as you raise the shoulder blades from the floor.

- Keep the movement slow and controlled in both the lifting and the lowering phase of the exercise.

- Be careful not to over-rotate. You are turning the shoulders just enough to engage the muscles around your waist. If you can feel them working, then you are rotating far enough.

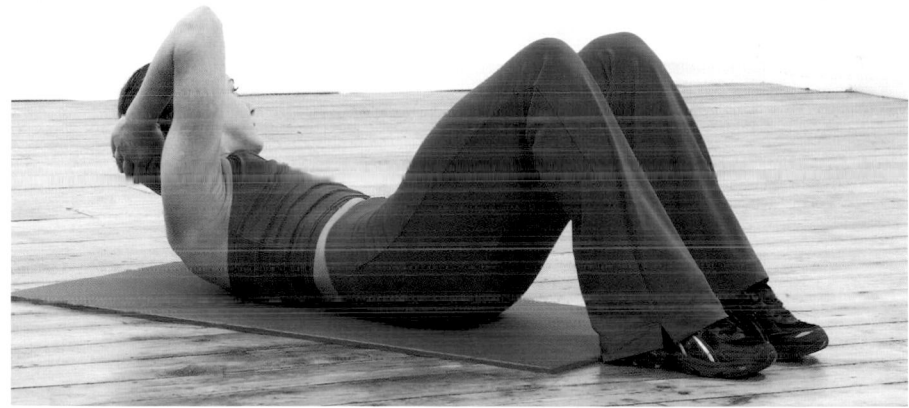

2 Curl up, lifting your shoulder blade off the floor, and rotate the upper body to one side while keeping your lower back and feet in contact with the floor.

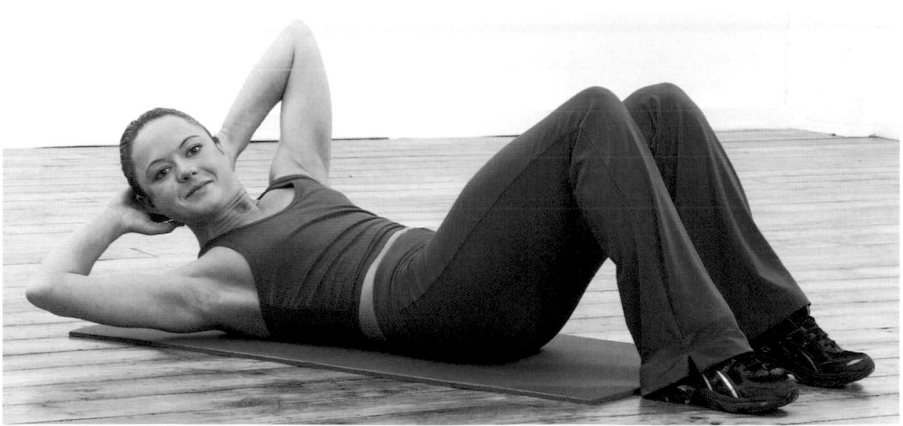

3 Slowly lower back down, leaving a small gap between the floor and your upper back and repeat the movement, this time rotating the upper body in the opposite direction. Continue the exercise, alternating the direction the torso rotates.

Abs/Back—Beginners

reverse curl

Area Worked: Front of stomach (lower).
Name of Muscle: Rectus Abdominus.

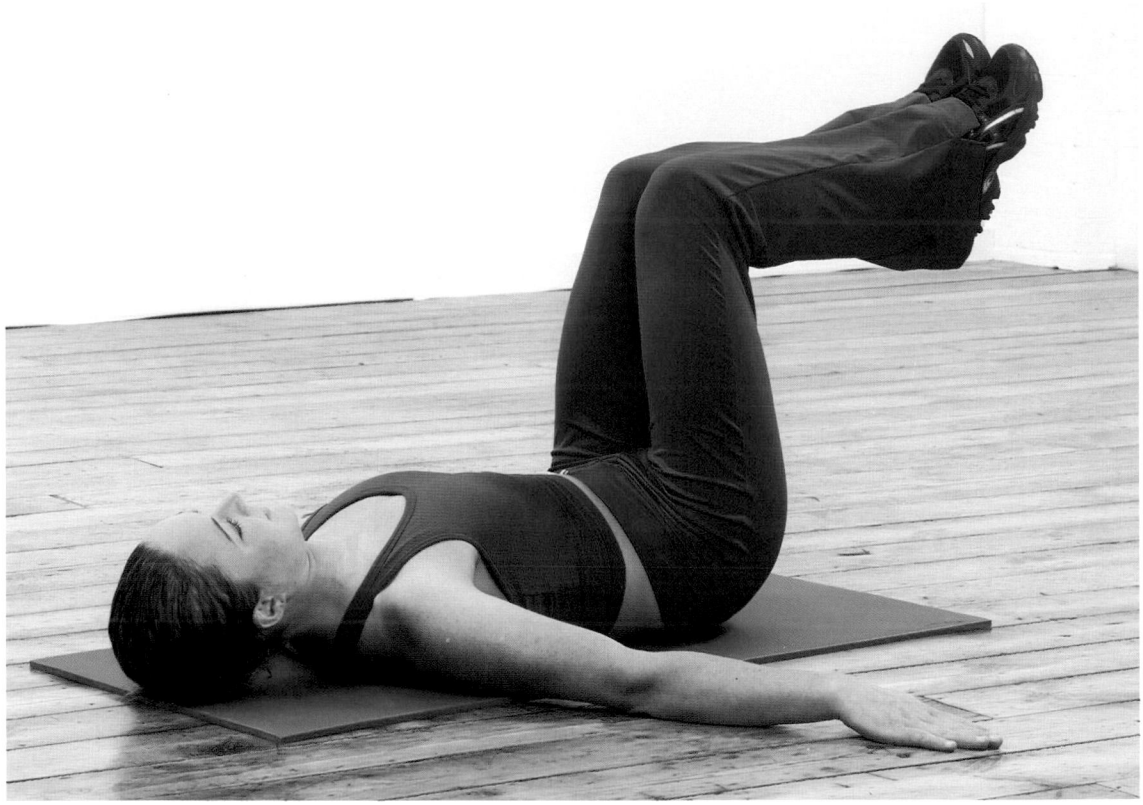

1 Lie on your back with your knees bent, feet flat on the floor, and your hands on the floor by your sides to stabilize you. Lift your feet off the floor so that your thighs are vertical and your knees are still bent.

Hints & Tips

• The stronger your muscles becomet, the straighter you can make your legs, but be careful as this puts pressure on your lower back. If you feel your lower back start to arch, then your abdominal muscles have done as much as they can.

Technique

- Keep your neck relaxed and your head on the floor throughout the exercise.

- Fix the knees at a 90-degree bend and think about moving through an arc with the feet.

- When curling the knees, pull the abdominal muscles in and keep it slow. Try not to swing the legs in and out. Use the muscle.

- It is only a slight raise (approximately an inch or two) of the butt and hips from the floor.

- Your lower back should stay in contact with the floor at all times.

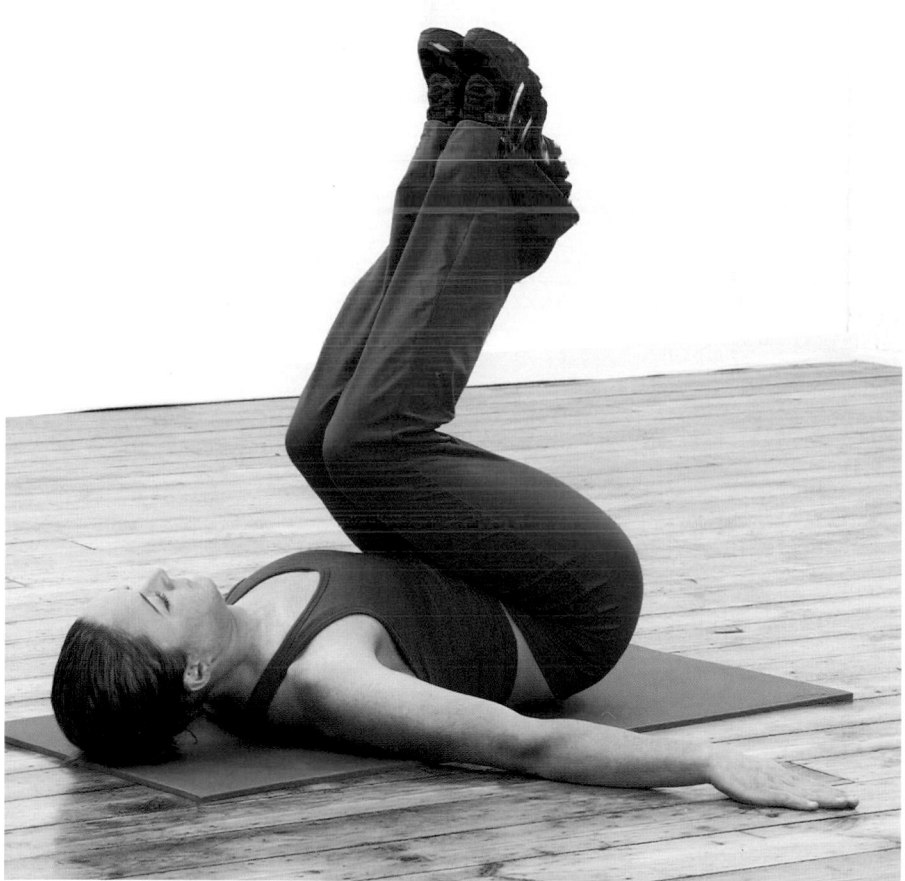

2 Lift your knees up and in as if you are bringing them to your chest and partially lift your butt off the floor. Slowly lower them back down to the start position, so that the thighs are again vertical.

Abs/Back—Beginners

alternating superman

Area Worked: Lower back.
Name of Muscle: Erector Spinae.

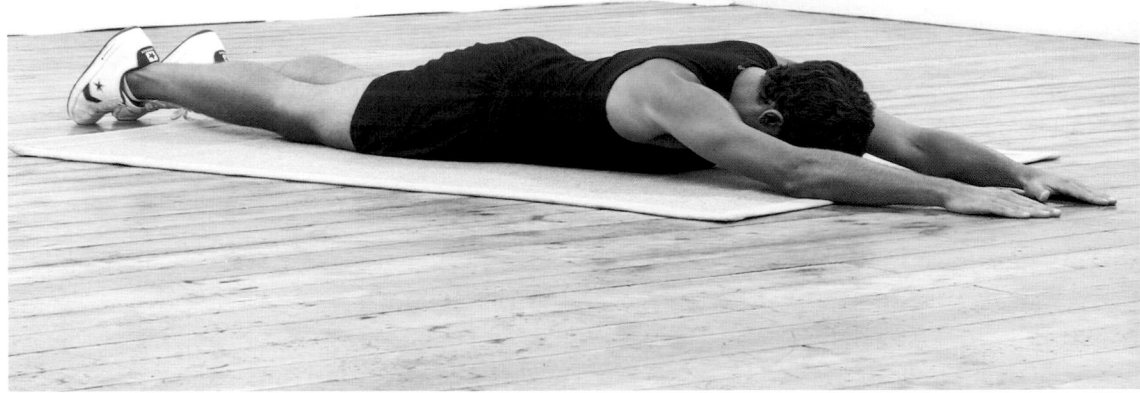

1 Lay face down on the floor with your legs out behind and your arms out in front.

Hints & Tips

• The movement is small but that doesn't mean that you have to rush through it. The movement should be a slow and gradual process. You should feel a gradual tightening of the muscle that you are working and then a slow release of that tightness as you lower back down.

Technique

- Keep a slight bend in the knees and elbows during the exercise.

- Always look at the floor. Try not to look up, as this will put strain on the back of your neck.

- Keep the movement small. Your body is not designed to move very far in this direction so try not to force it. You are trying to feel for a tightening of the muscles in your lower back.

2 Keeping the chest and the hips on the floor, raise the opposite arm and the opposite leg. Slowly lower them back to the floor and repeat on the other side.

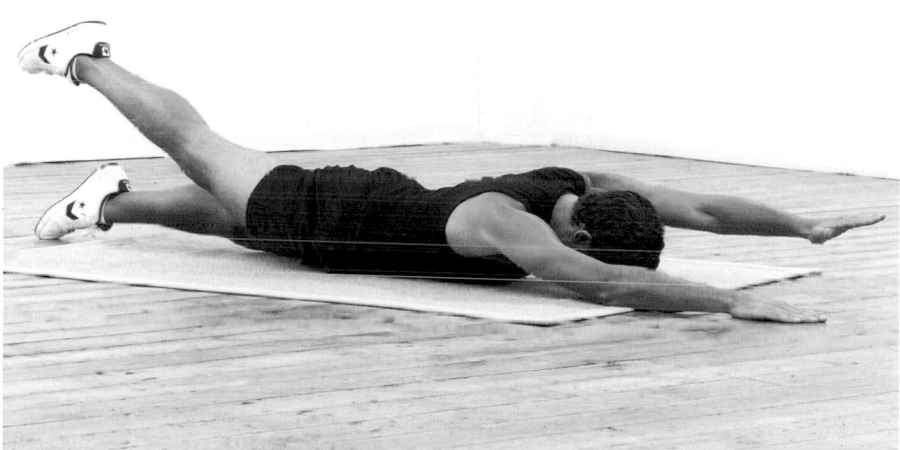

3 Continue the set by alternating the movement with each repetition.

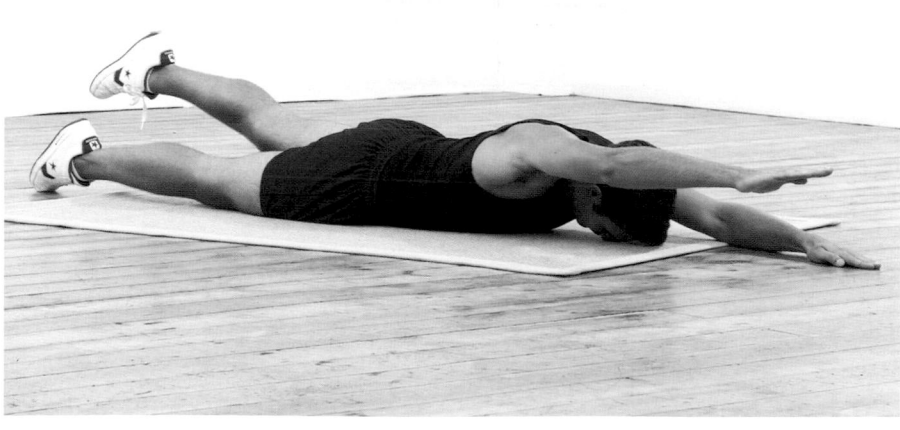

Abs/Back–Advanced

full bridge

Area Worked: Stomach.
Name of Muscles: Transverse Abdominus and Rectus Abdominus.

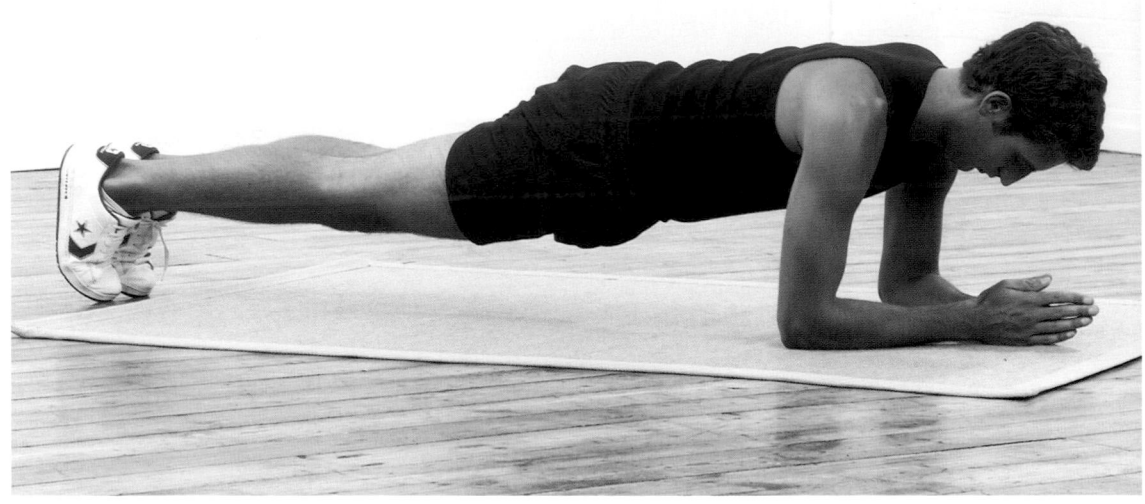

1 Walk the knees back until you have a straight line through your shoulders, hips, and knees. Maintaining the position of your torso, raise the knees from the floor.

Hints & Tips

- Do not hold your breath. It is a natural outcome when holding this position that you may find it difficult to breathe. Focus on holding your position and keep your stomach pulled in.

- If you do have difficulty, practice standing up. Turn sideways in front of a mirror and suck your stomach in. Now focus on keeping it there while you breathe in and out. You should see your ribcage moving as your lungs inhale and exhale, but your stomach should stay put.

Technique

- Keep your elbows below your shoulders, make your hands into fists and bring them together to make a triangle. You should feel stable in this position.

- Keep the knees the same width apart as your hips during the exercise.

- Be careful not to let your hips drop toward the floor. Keep your abdominal muscles pulled in tight.

- Do not push your butt in the air. You should have a straight line from shoulders to feet.

2 Hold this position. You will know for how long, when the desire to drop the hips becomes too much.

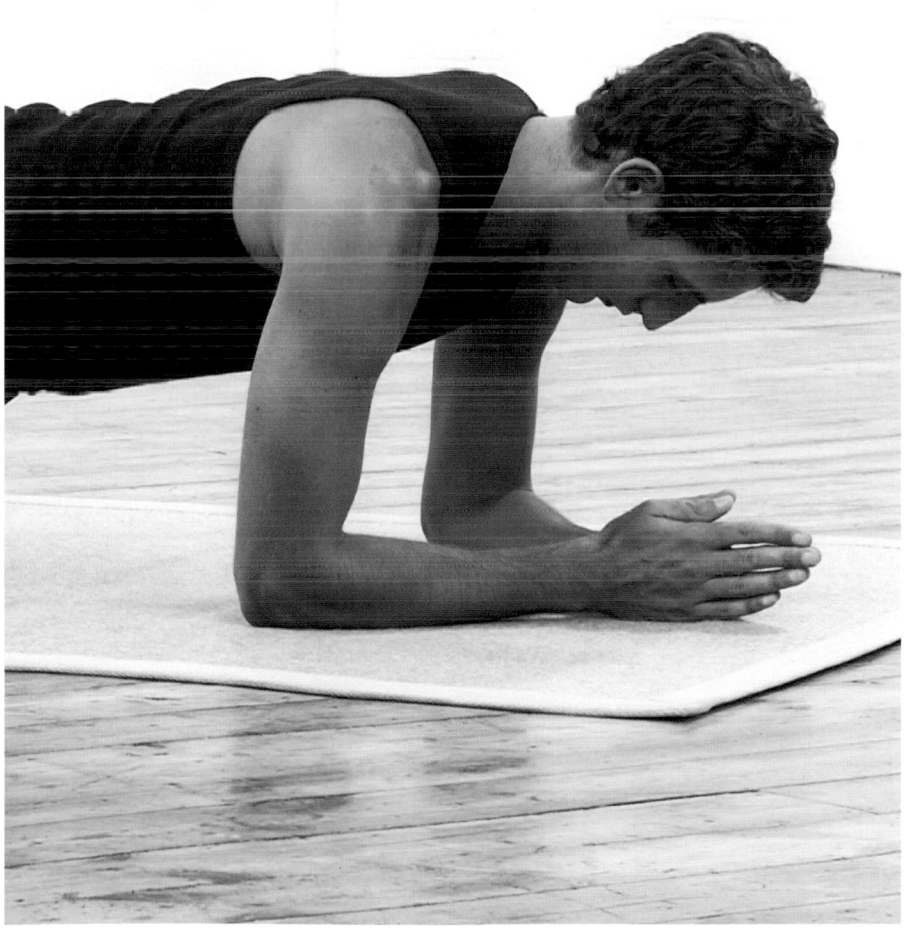

Abs/Back–Advanced

abdominal crunch

Area Worked: Front of stomach (upper).
Name of Muscle: Rectus Abdominus.

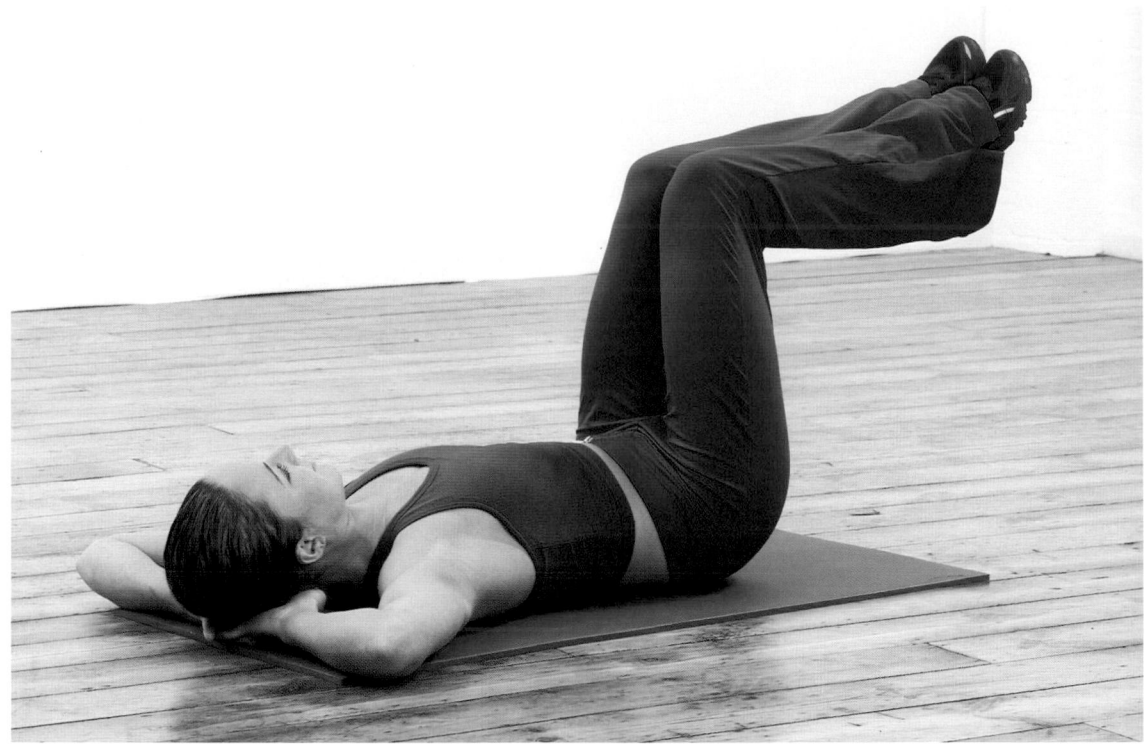

1 Lay on your back with your knees bent and your feet flat on the floor. Lift the knees and feet up so that you have a 90-degree angle at the hips and the same at the knees.

Hints & Tips

• Engage the muscles as if you were going to pull your knees in toward your chest but do not physically move them. This should help to keep your stomach pulled in.

Technique

- Pull your abdominal muscles in as you curl up.

- Keep a small gap, approximately the size of your fist, between your chin and your chest and try not to push your head forward as you curl up.

- You only need to lift a few inches from the floor.

- Fix your legs in one position. Your butt should still be on the floor as you lift up.

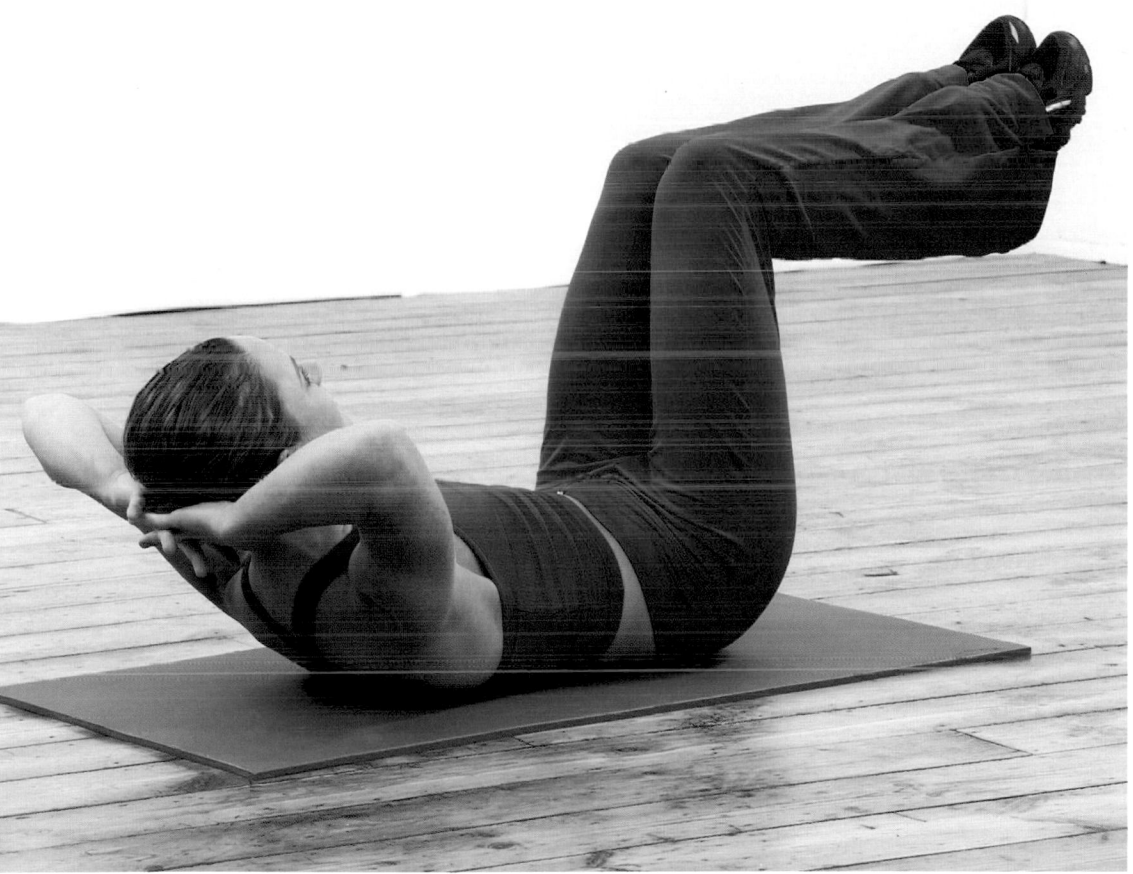

2 Curl up, lifting your shoulder blades off the floor while keeping your lower back and feet in contact with the floor. Slowly lower down, leaving a small gap between the floor and your upper back, and repeat the movement.

Abs/Back—Advanced

rotating side bridge

Area Worked: Sides of stomach (waist).
Name of Muscles: Obliques.

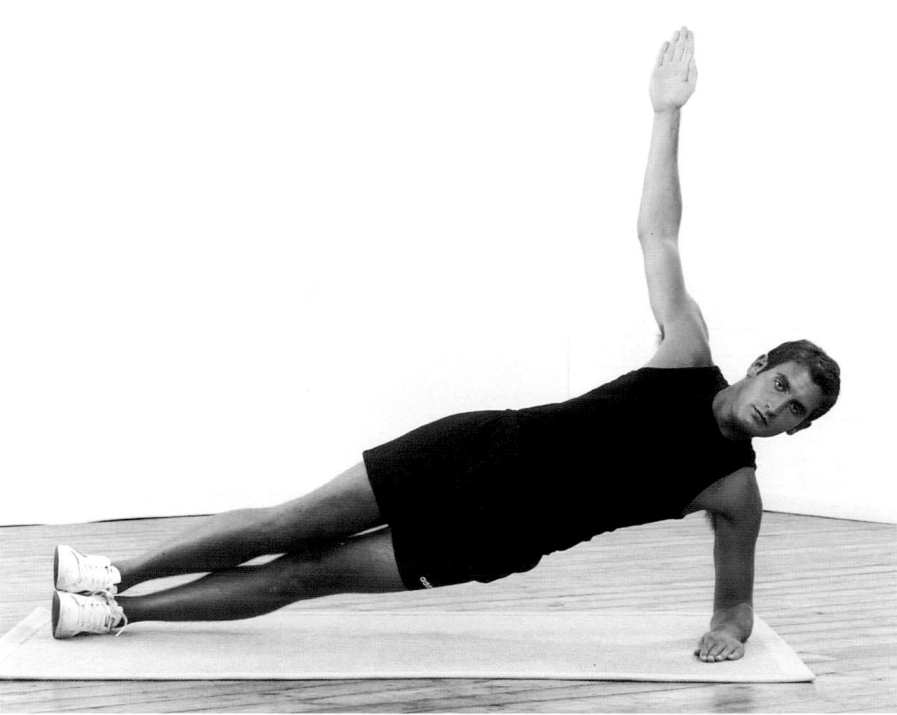

1 Lie on your side with your weight resting on your elbow. Keeping the body straight, lift your hip from the floor so that your weight is now supported on your feet and your elbow.

Hints & Tips

• Keep the abdominal muscles pulled in, and your hip pushed high all the way through the exercise to help with your balance.

• As you become more proficient, try holding a light weight in your hand. But remember not to swing. Be slow and controlled to work those muscles to the full.

Technique

- Keep the weight on your elbow and forearm. Your forearm should point the same way that you are looking.

- Your body should be straight from head to toe.

- Keep a slight bend in the elbow of the free arm during the movement.

- Focus on keeping the hips still during the rotation. The movement should come from around your waist with your hips pointing forward.

- Stack the feet one on top of the other. This may take practice but will become easier

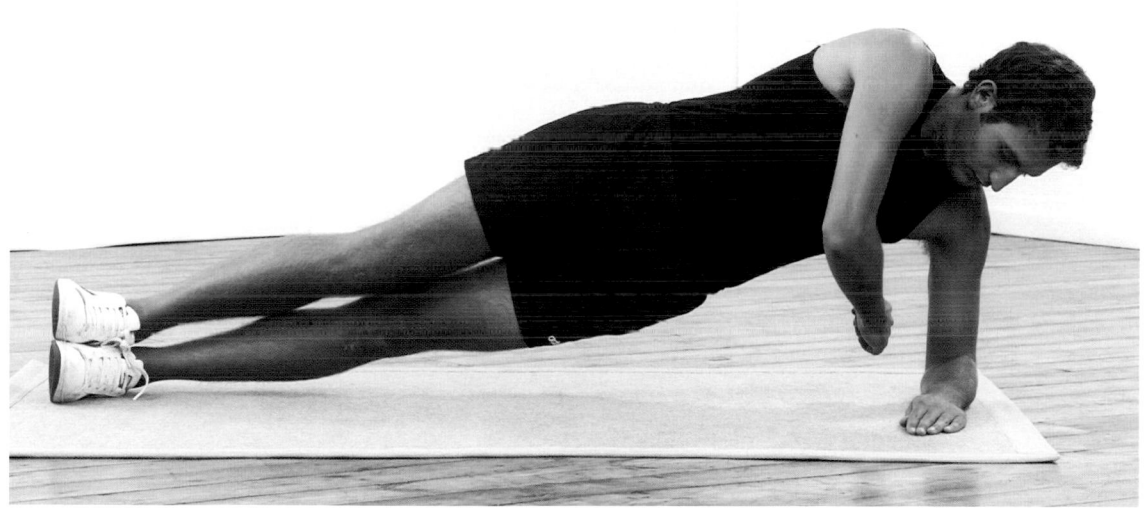

2 Place the free hand straight up in to the air and in one smooth movement rotate the upper body and reach underneath to the opposite elbow. Going through the same range of movement, place the hand back in the air and repeat for the set number of repetitions, before doing the same on the other side.

Abs/Back–Advanced

heel drops

Area Worked: Front of stomach and hips.
Name of Muscles: Transverse Abdominus and Hip Flexor.

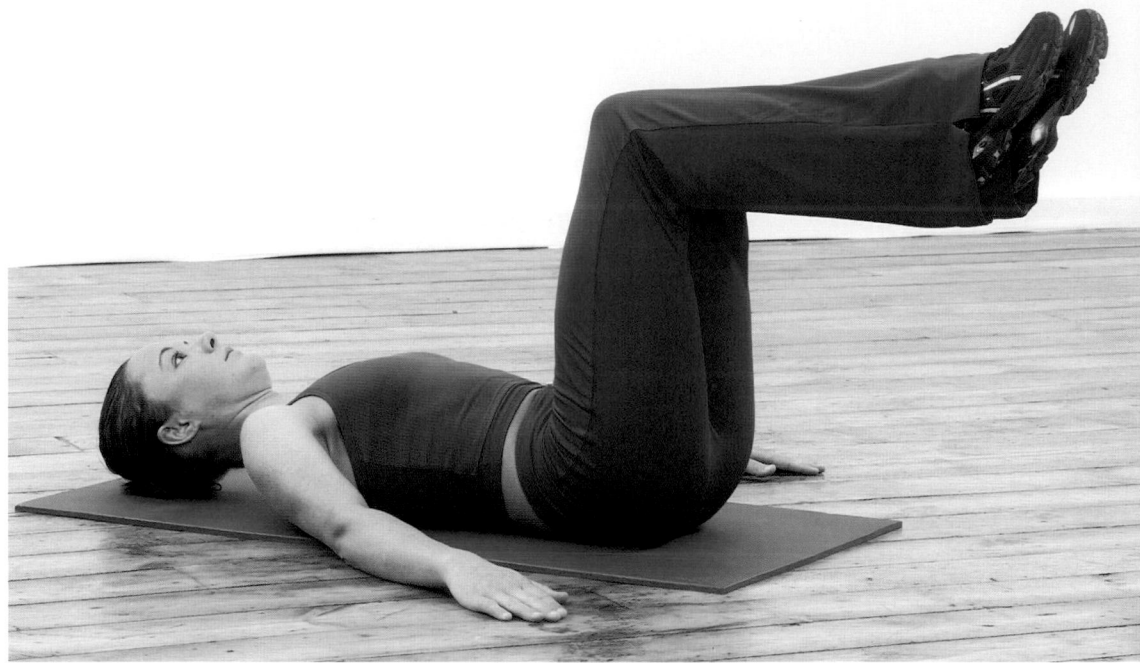

1 Lie on your back with your hands by your sides and your legs raised in the air with a slight bend in the knee. Keeping one leg where it is, lower the other leg down until the heel is just above the floor.

Hints & Tips

• When you have paused at the bottom, just before you start to lift, pull in your abdominal muscles and keep pulling all the way to the top. Follow this process for each repetition. Pause, pull, lift ...

Technique

- Keep the neck relaxed with the head on the floor. Brace the abs to keep your back in contact with the floor.

- Lower slowly and lift even more slowly. Lift too quickly and the muscle you are targeting does not need to work as hard.

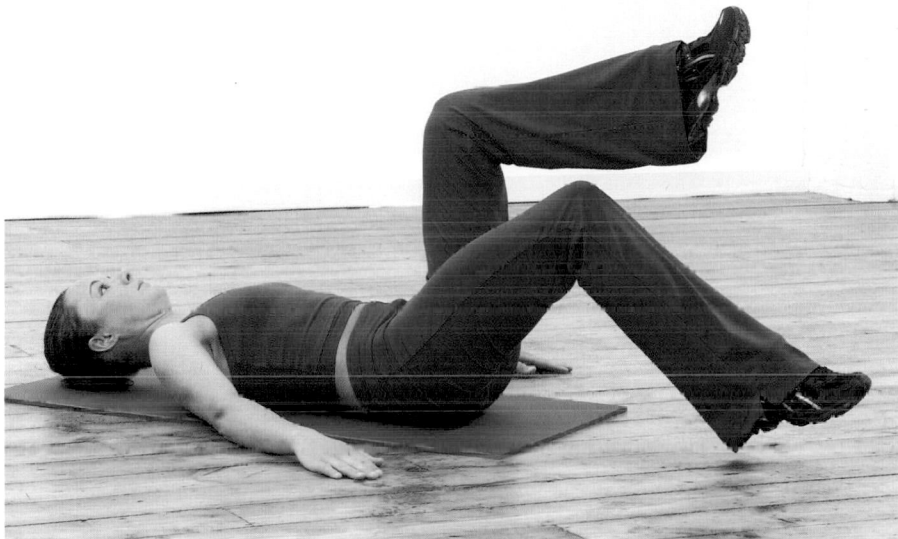

2 Pause for a second and then return to the start position.

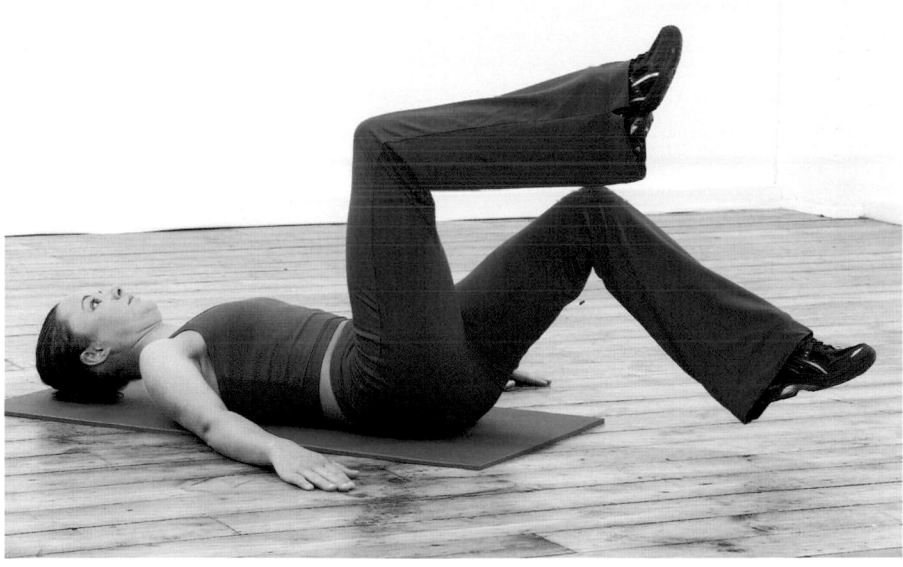

3 Repeat the movement with the other leg and continue the set by alternating the legs on each repetition.

Abs/Back–Advanced

back extension

Area Worked: Lower back.
Name of Muscles: Erector Spinae.

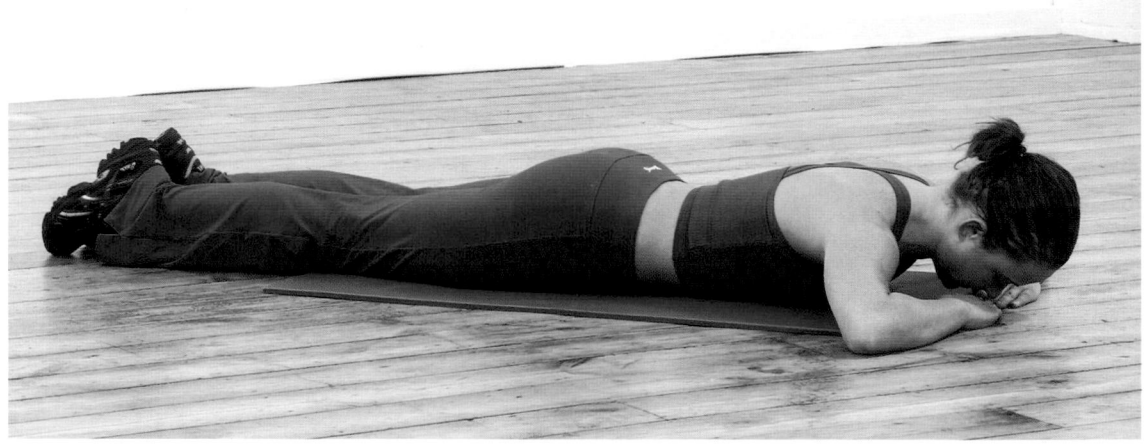

1 Lie face down on the floor with your legs straight out behind you and your fingertips at your temples.

Hints & Tips

- The movement is small, so as long as you can feel the muscles in your lower back tighten as you lift, that will be high enough.

- Remember that the floor in front of you has suddenly become the most interesting thing in the world until you have finished your set.

Technique

- Try to keep your butt and legs relaxed during the movement. You will know when you are doing this because your knees and toes will stay on the floor.

- Always look at the floor as you lift up. This will keep the strain off your neck and help to keep your spine in alignment.

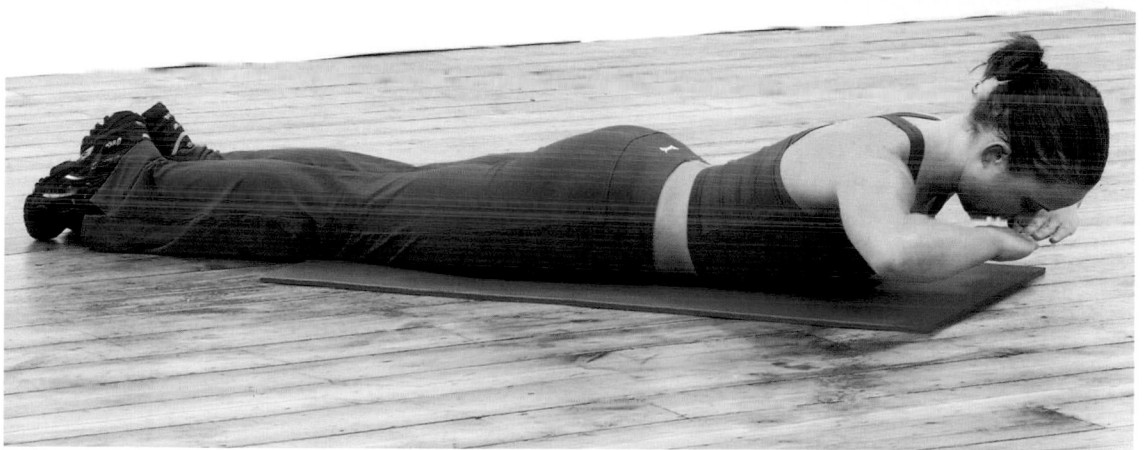

2 Slowly lift your chest from the floor and slowly lower back down. Do not completely rest at the bottom and repeat the movement.

Whole Body–Advanced

deadlift

Area Worked: Thighs, butt, lower and upper back.
Name of Muscles: Quads, Hamstrings, Gluteus, Erector Spinae, Latissimus Dorsi, Trapezius.

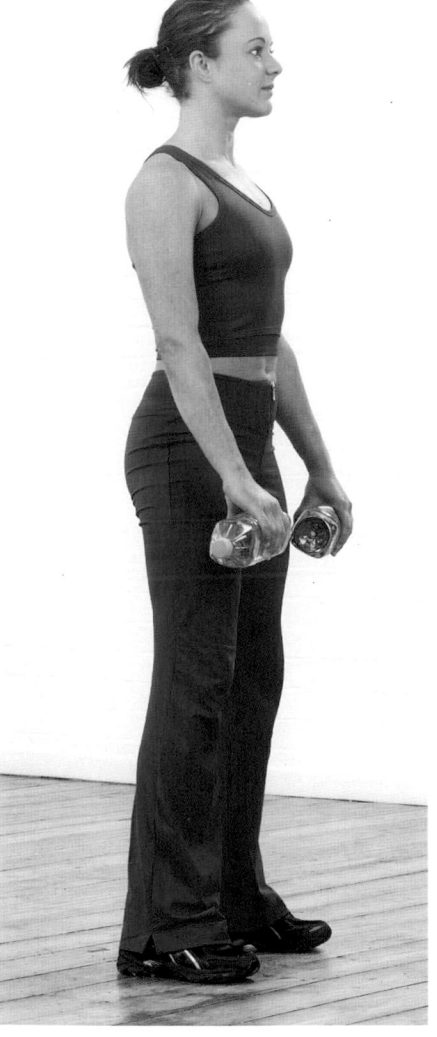

The following three exercises combine to form an exercise called the Clean and Press. You will have seen the exercise before if you watch weightlifting. It is an exercise where a weight is lifted from the floor and up to the top of the chest where the weight rests. The weight is then pushed, using both the lower and the upper body, over the head. It is a powerful movement utilizing almost all the major muscle groups, while also requiring a lot of timing and muscle coordination.

Remember: the Deadlift is the technique you should use whenever you lift any weight from the floor.

1 Stand tall, holding a weight in each hand in front of your thighs.

Hints & Tips

• The movement and technique is very similar to the Weighted Squat, except the weights are in front of you rather than at the side. This means that you have to consciously tip forward while maintaining your posture. More work therefore has to be done by the muscles through the back.

• Start light and focus on your lifting technique rather than the weight itself. This is an exercise where once you have confidence in your technique you can advance very quickly on the amount of weight lifted.

Technique

- Because the weights are in front of your thighs, be sure to focus on pulling your shoulders back to counteract the tendency to round the back.

- Keep the weights in front of you at all times. They should stay as close to your body as you can get them, without hitting your knees as you lower them down.

- Just before you start to lower the weights, follow this mental check list: chest lifted, abdominals braced, hips back.

- Reverse this process for lifting back up and, like the Squat, try to keep your weight on your heels.

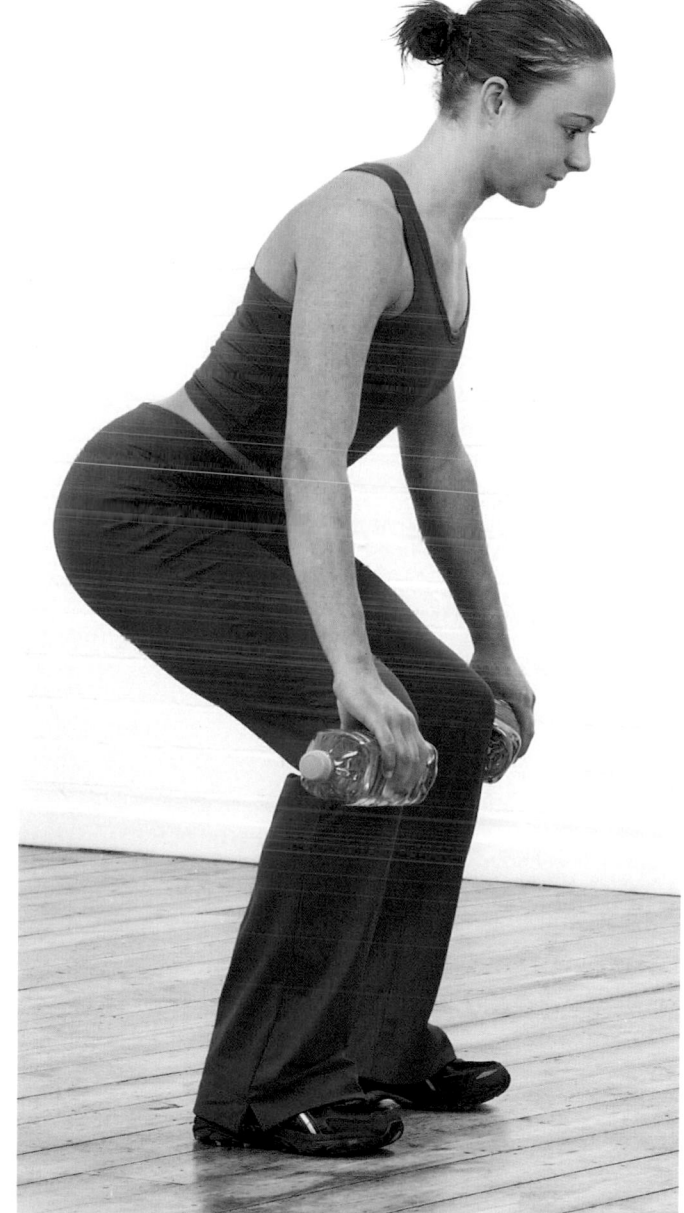

2 Keeping the chest lifted, push the hips back and bend the knees, lowering the weights toward the floor. Push up, lifting the chest so that you return back to the starting position.

Whole Body–Advanced

clean

Area Worked: As for the Deadlift, plus shoulders and front of arms.
Name of Muscles: As for the Deadlift, plus Deltoids and Biceps.

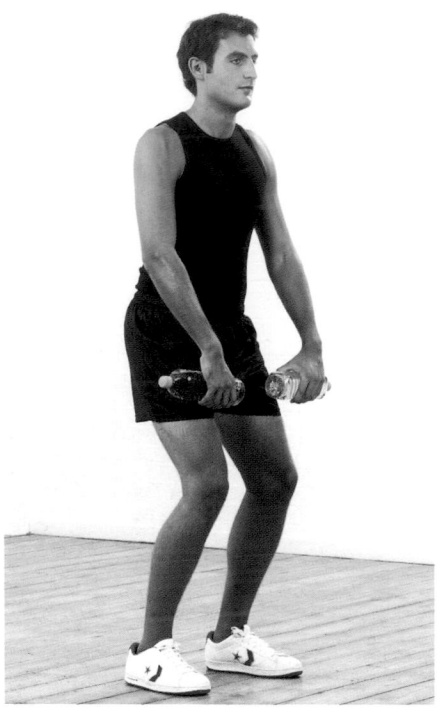 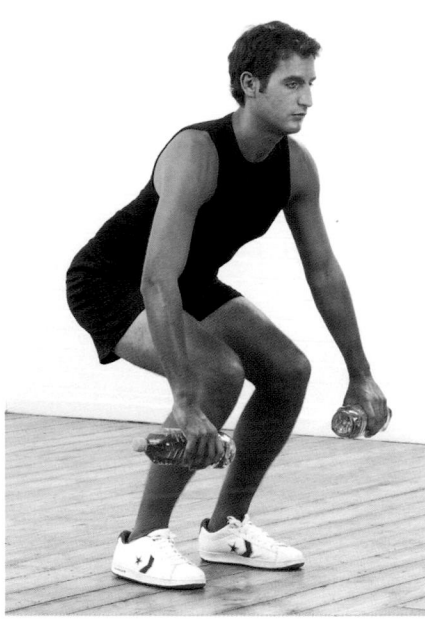

1 Stand tall, holding a weight in each hand in front of your thighs.

2 Keeping the chest lifted, push the hips back and bend the knees, lowering the weights toward the floor.

Hints & Tips

• Your legs have the strongest muscles in your body. Use them to power the weight up and use the momentum that they generate to get the weights to your shoulders.

• When lowering the weights, remember to roll the wrists forward first and then roll the elbows up to keep the tension in your shoulders without strain.

Technique

- Follow the Deadlift technique and then add the following.

- You are focussing on powering the legs up as quickly as you can to generate momentum, so that the movement is then continued by the arms when they pull the weight up to the chest.

- Keep the weights close to the body throughout the lift at approximately shoulder-width.

- Focus on keeping the elbows high.

- As the weights reach approximately chest height, start to bend the knees slightly as if

moving underneath the weight, which you should still be pulling up.

- Roll the elbows underneath and let the wrists follow so that the weights are now sitting at shoulder height. Your elbows should be underneath the weights with your palms forward, your knuckles facing the ceiling, and the knees soft.

- When returning the weight back down, start by rolling the wrists forward and then rotate the arms over the top of the weights. Your elbows should now be slightly higher than the weights before you lower them again.

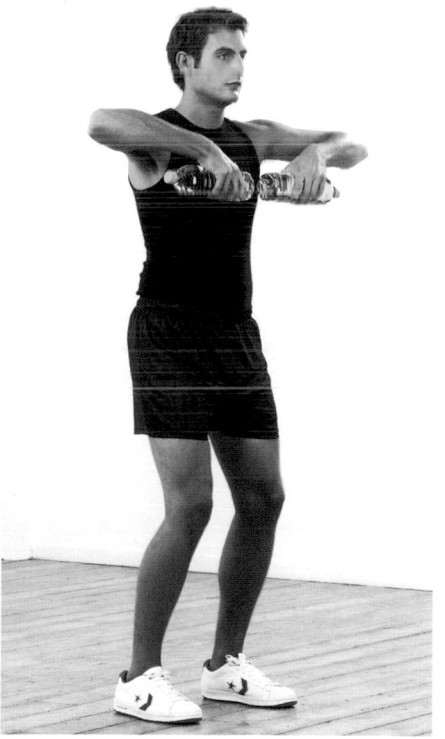

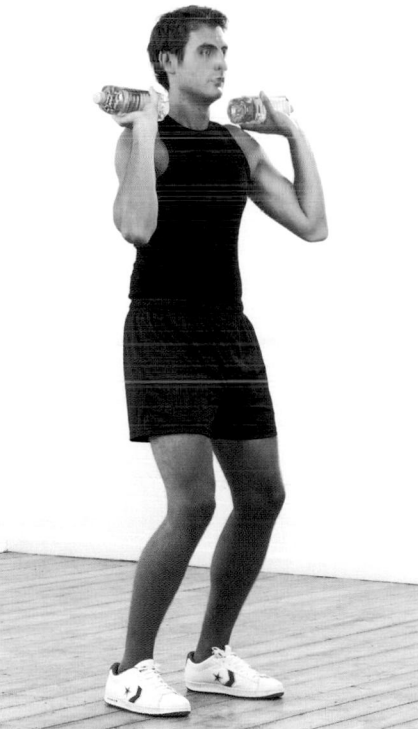

3 Push from the bottom of the movement, lifting the chest. As the legs straighten, pull the weights up in front of you.

4 When the weights reach your chest soften the knees again and roll the elbows underneath so that the weights are now at shoulder height, with the palms facing forward and the knuckles facing the ceiling.

Whole Body—Advanced

shoulder push press

Area Worked: Thighs, shoulders, and back of the arms.
Name of Muscles: Quadriceps, Hamstrings, Deltoids, and Triceps.

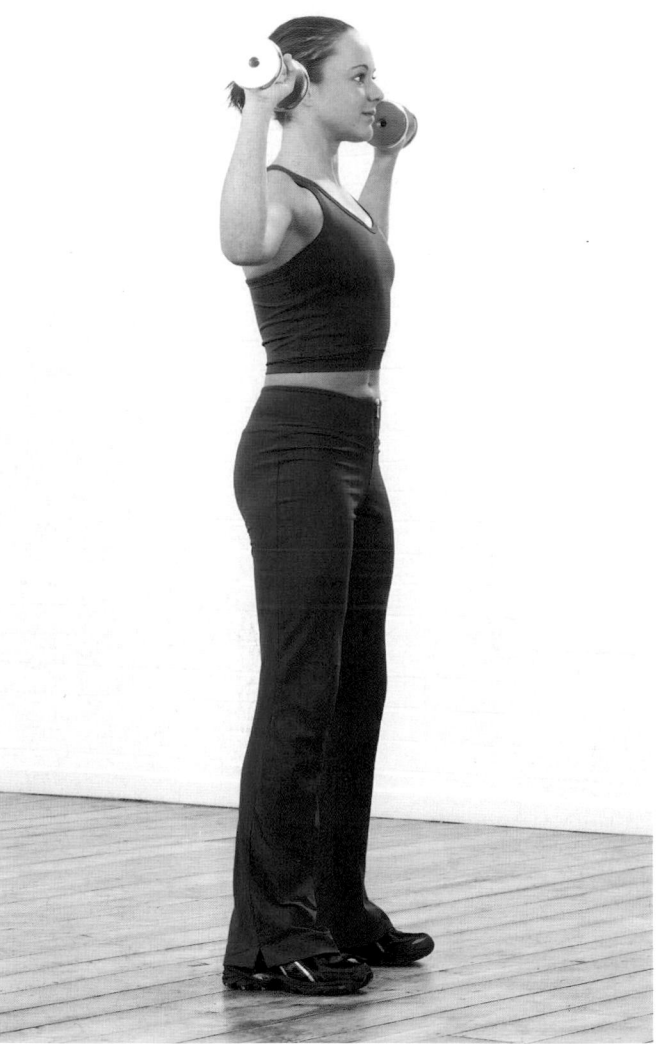

1 Start with the weights by your shoulders. Your knuckles should face the ceiling with your palms forward. Your elbows should be pointing to the floor below the weights. This is the top position of the "Clean" exercise.

Hints & Tips

- When you move from your slightly squat position and push with the legs there will be a point when the weights in your hand feel light. This is the point at which you start to push with your hands to keep the momentum generated by your legs going.

Technique

- Keep the abdominal muscles braced to maintain correct posture, which is the key to this exercise.

- When bending the knees, remember to tilt the pelvis and push the hips back. How low you go will depend on how heavy the weight is. The heavier the weight, the more help you will need from your legs as

these are a much stronger muscle than your shoulders. Your legs will help to push the weight up along with the shoulders, so really power the legs up when you straighten them.

- When you do straighten the legs and the arms remember not to lock them out. Keep the joints straight, but soft.

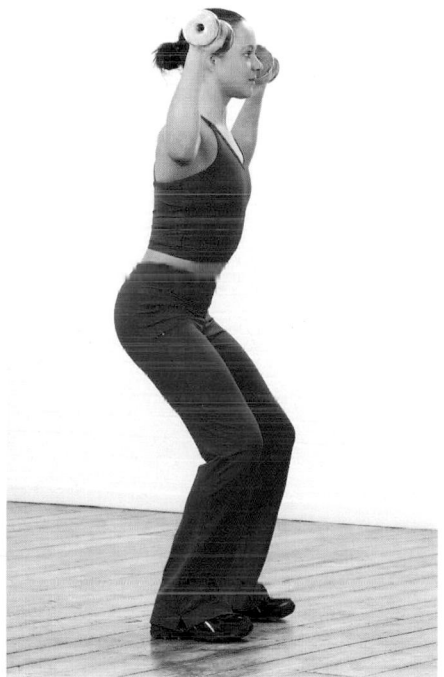

2 Bend the knees slightly, as if you were about to start a squat.

3 Quickly straighten the legs and push the weights up over the head. Lower the weights back down to the starting position, at the same time bending the knees slightly.

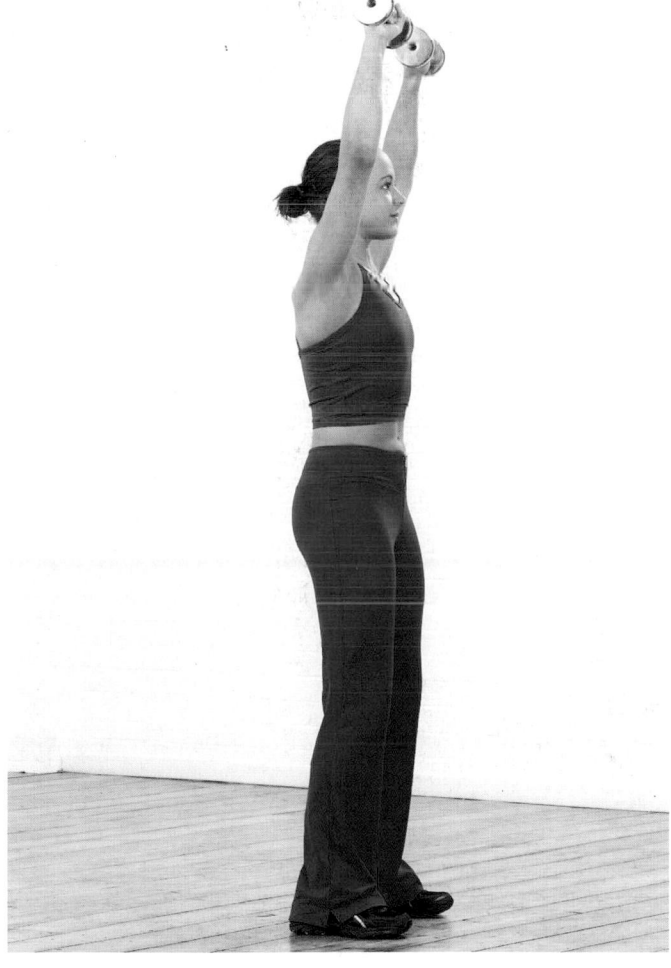

Whole Body—Advanced

clean and press

Area Worked: Thighs, butt, lower and upper back, shoulders, back and front of the arms.
Name of Muscles: As for the Clean and Shoulder Push Press combined.

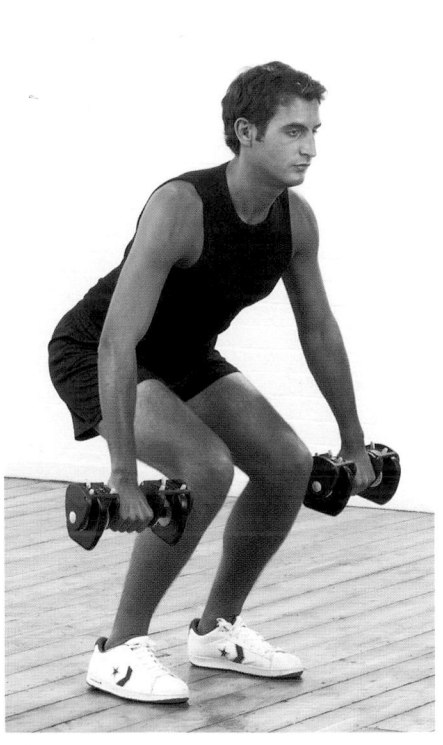
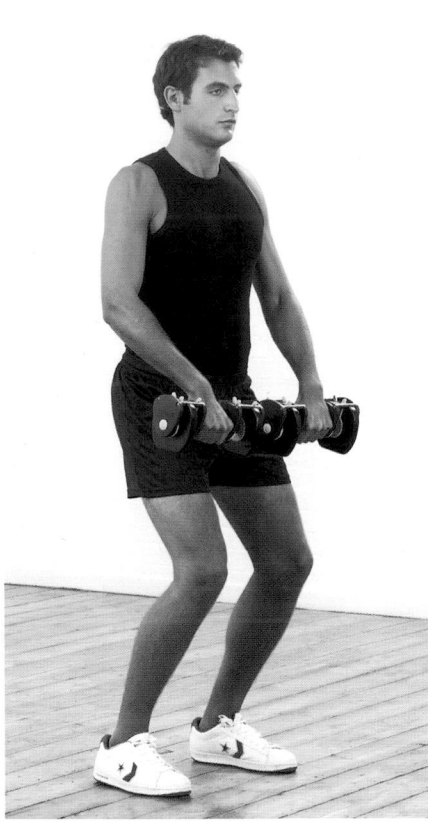

1 This is a combination of the Clean and the Shoulder Push Press. Stage one is the clean to get the weights from the floor up to the shoulders.

Hints & Tips

• Obviously, the common-sense approach is to practice the Clean and the Shoulder Push Press as two distinct exercises before trying the Clean and Press.

Technique

- See the technique points for the Clean and the Shoulder Push Press.

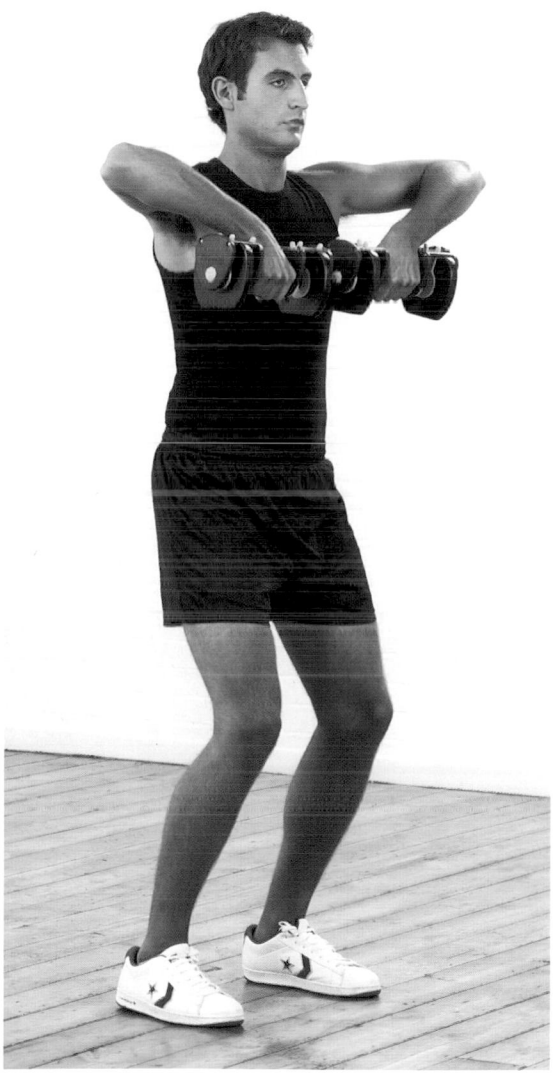 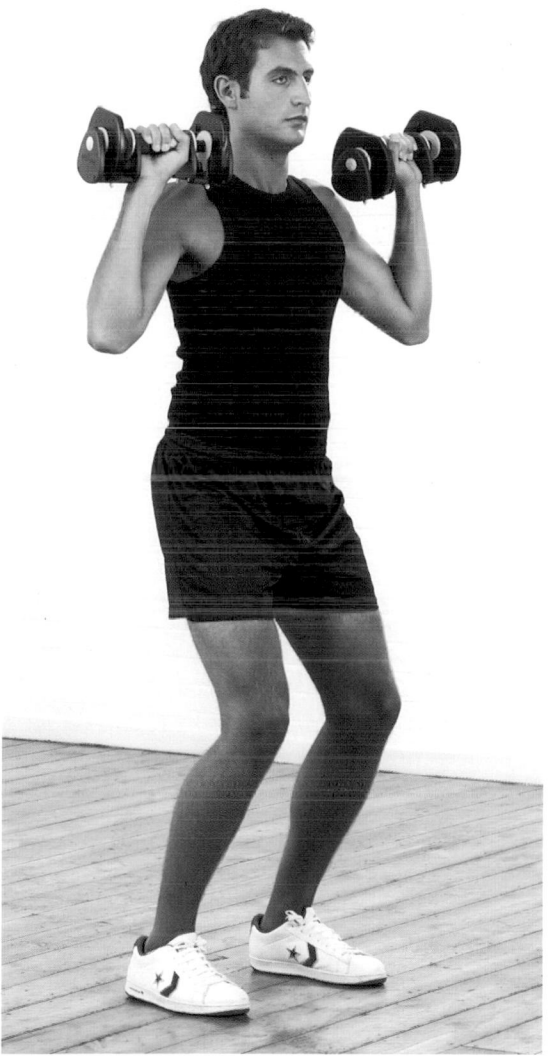

2 Stage two is the Shoulder Push Press to lift the weights from the shoulders to above the head.

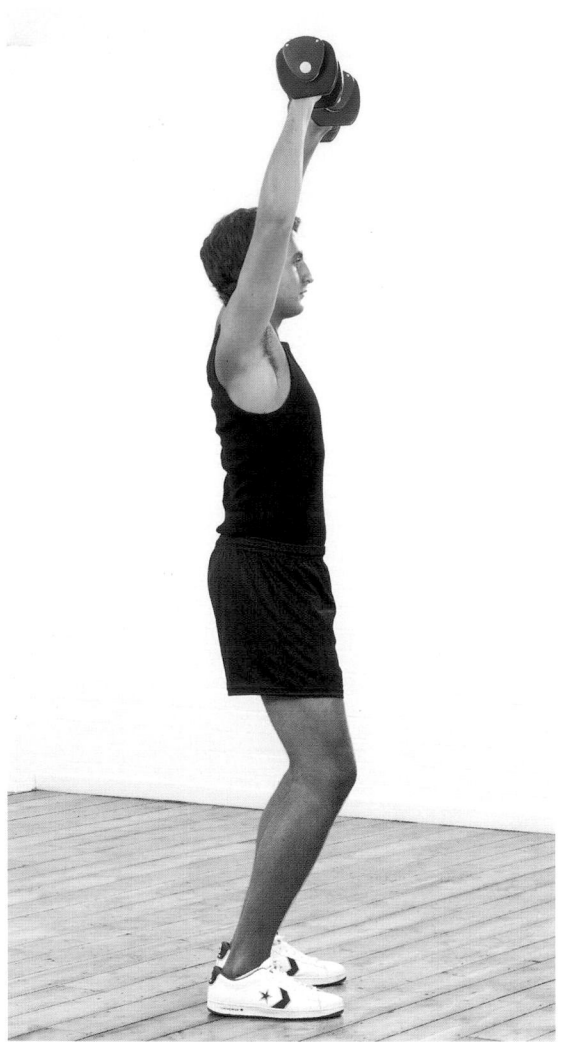
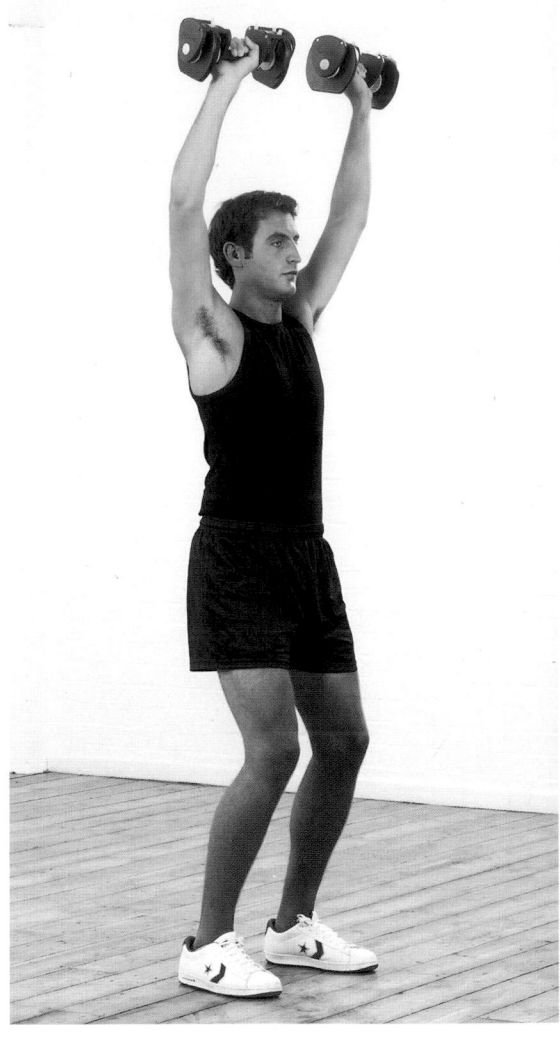

3 The process is then reversed. The weights come from over the head back to the shoulders. They are then rolled and lowered down the front of the body and back down towards the floor.

4 Neither the knee nor the elbow joints are locked, even at the top of the movement.

The Workouts

We are now going to put those exercises from the previous sections into several different workouts, each with a specific aim. The workouts last approximately 20 minutes with a light warm-up, warm-down, and stretch (see Pre and Post-Workout, page 15, for details).
Initially it may be that workouts last longer but as you become more familiar with the exercises and the order that they are in, you will find that they will easily fit in to that 20-minute time slot. Showering is not included in that time but is recommended!
The workouts can be done in any order you like, but initially it is recommended that you follow them in the order that they are set, as they are designed gradually to introduce different principles as the weeks progress. These start with familiarizing you with some of the exercises before gradually increasing the intensity and the variety in the routines. The table below shows how to follow the workouts over several weeks. Enjoy!

Workout Name	Duration	Frequency	Notes
Basic Workout	3–4 weeks	2–3 times/week (non consecutive days)	Focuses on technique and familiarizing yourself with regular exercise.
Two-Day Upper/Lower Split	4–6 weeks	2–4 times/week	Introduces a greater variety of exercises. Aims to gradually increase intensity over workouts.
Two-Day Push/Pull Split	4–6 weeks	2–4 times/week	Introduces new exercises. Builds intensity as weeks progress.
Superset Circuit	2–3 weeks	2–3 times/week (non consecutive days)	Increases intensity. A different type of training designed to increase calorie expenditure. Use as a variation on previous workouts.
Strength Workout	3–4 weeks	2–3 times/week (non consecutive days)	Focuses on increasing weight. A different type of training. Use as a variation on previous workouts.
Pre-fatigue Workout	3–6 weeks	2–3 times/week (non consecutive days)	Use as an alternative workout with weight as the limiting factor for increasing intensity.

Workout—Beginners

three sets

When in doubt, start here. Even when you have progressed beyond these basic exercises, you can return to this workout as an extended warm-up, or on days when you feel fragile.

The core workouts to focus on for most of the time are the Two-Day Upper/Lower Split and the Two-Day Push/Pull Split. These will work the most muscle groups with the greatest variety of exercise. The Basic Workout is there purely as an introduction to resistance training. As mentioned earlier, it takes time for your body to adapt to training, so the gentle approach is the best way to go. Lull that body into a false sense of security!

The latter three workouts are there to add variety. Once you have finished the first three cycles try the Superset Circuit for a change. Then go back to one of the Two-Day Splits. Then try the strength workout and back again to one of the Two-Day Splits. Keep the body guessing as to what is coming next.

Aims: To familiarize the individual with resistance training, focussing on correct technique. Attention should be paid to posture, recruiting the correct muscle in relation to the exercise, lifting and lowering speeds, and breathing.

Repetition Range: 10–15 repetitions. (Lifting two seconds. Lowering three+ seconds.)

Notes specific to workout: At this time do not worry about the amount of weight that you are lifting. Find a weight you feel confident with and one that you feel that you are in control of.

Rest after each set for between 30 seconds and one minute.

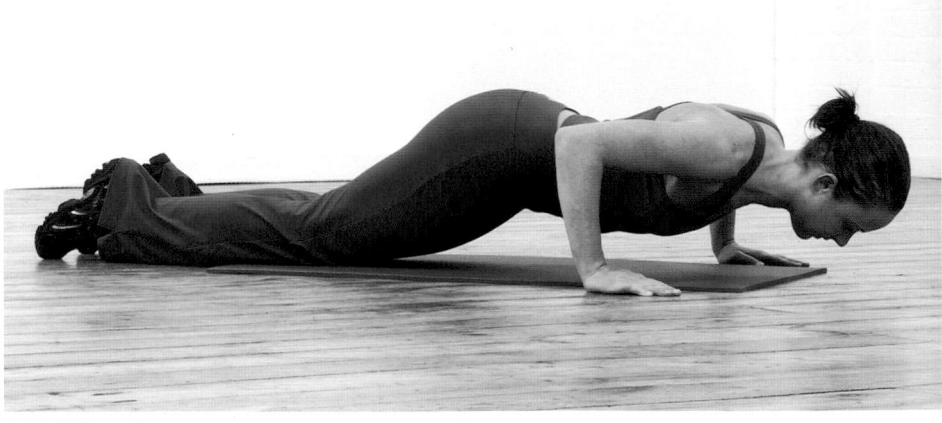

1 Half Press Up

Exercise Order

1 Half Press Up
2 Single Arm Row
3 Sit Down Squat
4 Shoulder Press
5 Half Bridge
6 Alternating Superman

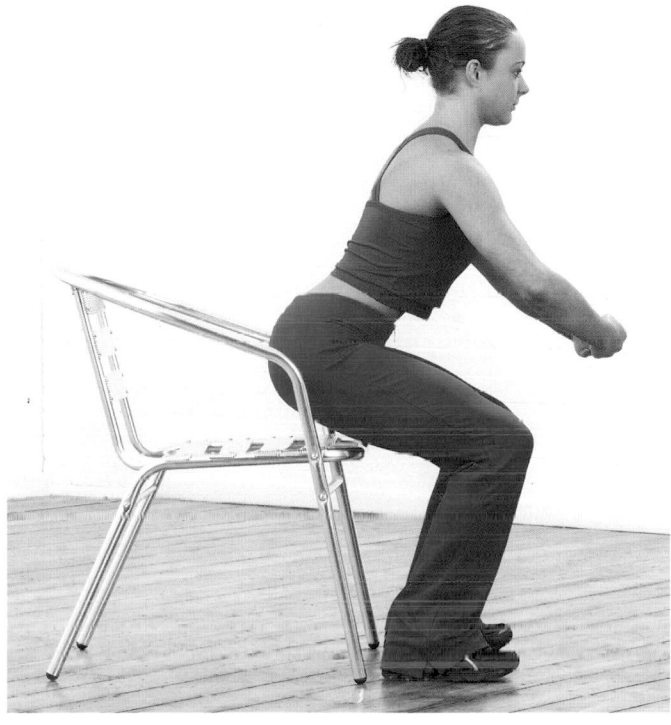

2 Single Arm Row

3 Sit Down Squat

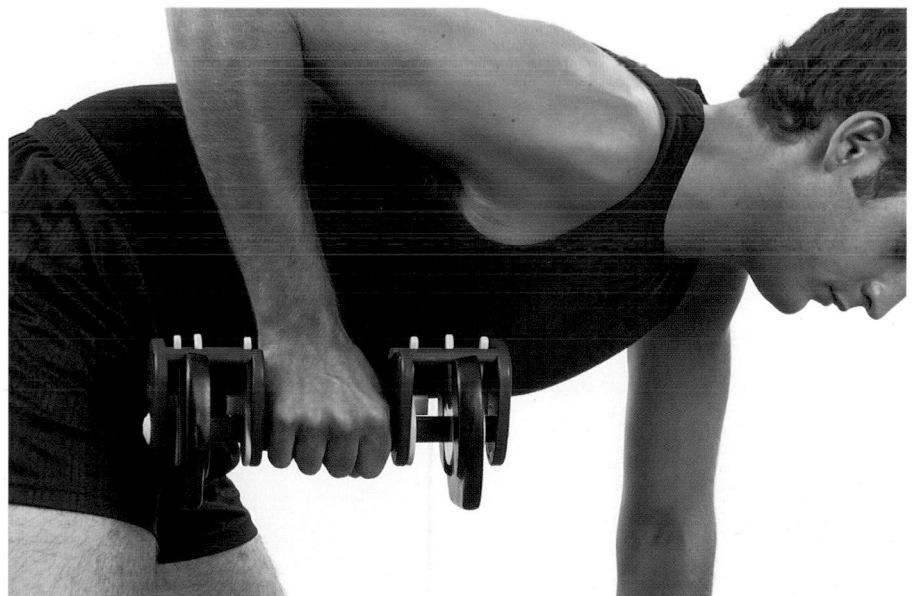

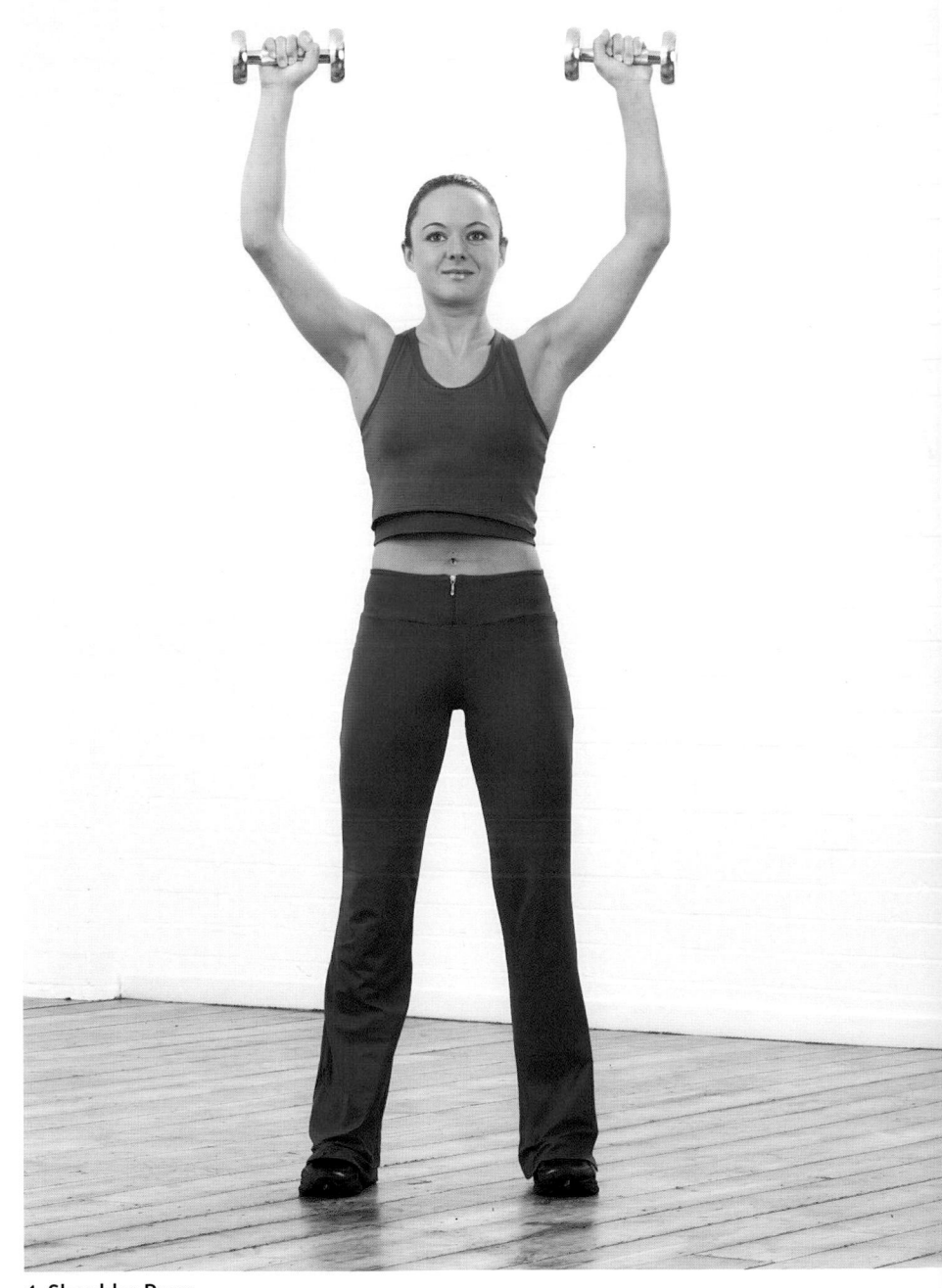

4 Shoulder Press

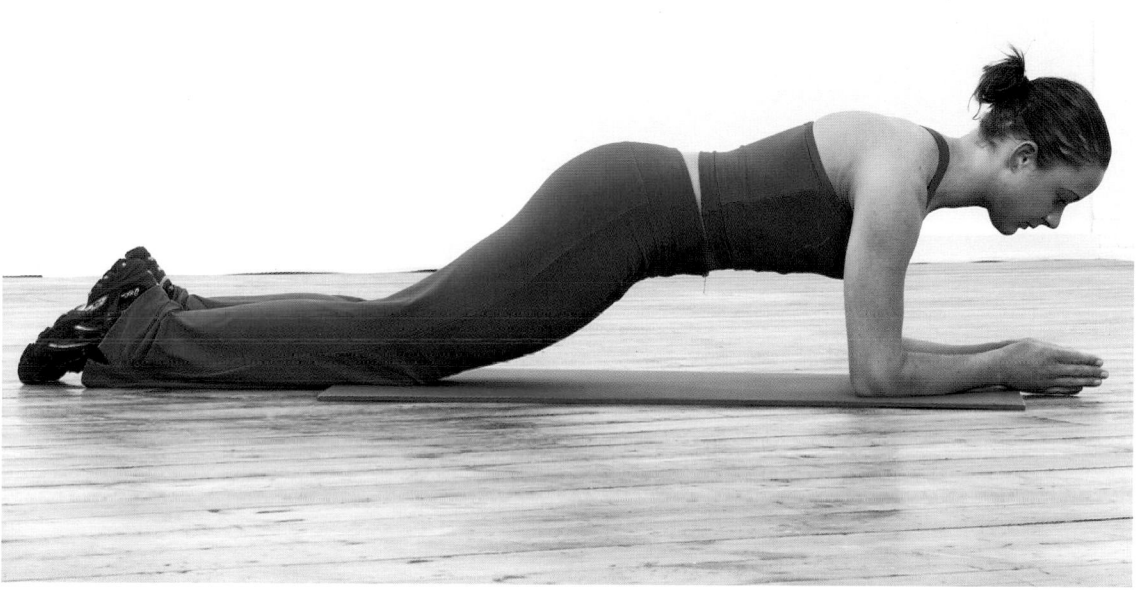

5 Half Bridge

6 Alternating Superman

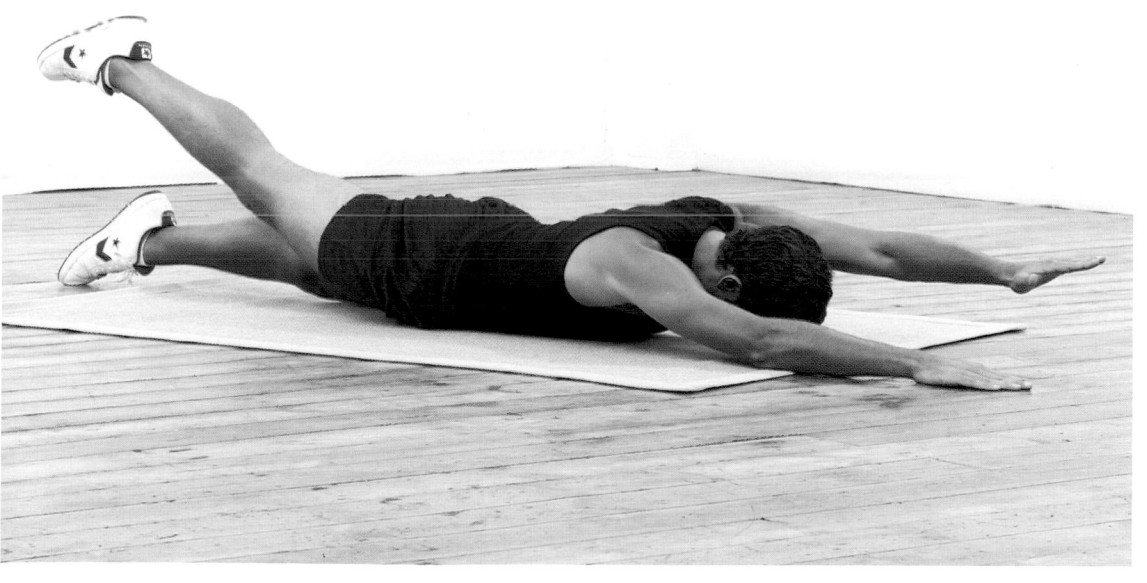

Body Split–Beginner

one set to near muscle fatigue

Splitting the body in two is a cunning way to force you back into your sneakers on two consecutive days.

Aims: To exercise a greater variety of muscles on separate days. One day to be spent concentrating on the upper body and one day on the lower body. While one set of muscles is working, the other muscles are resting, so that you can exercise on consecutive days.

Repetition Range: 10–15. (Lifting two seconds. Lowering three+ seconds.)

Notes specific to workout: Still focus on the technique, but aim to lift slightly heavier weights then you did in the base workout. You are only doing a single set so really focus on working hard. If you are getting to 15 repetitions and feel like you could do another three to five repetitions, then increase the weight. (The workouts include the abdominals and lower back in the lower body day).

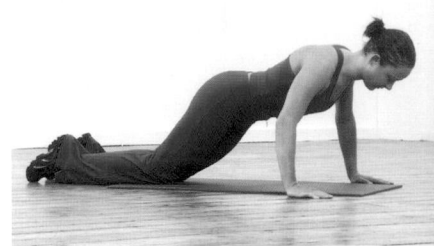

1 Half Press Up/Day 1

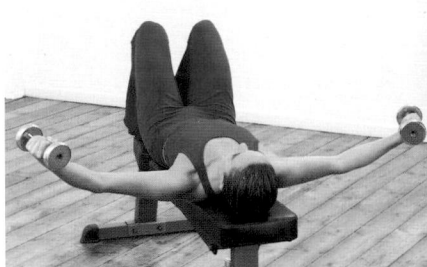

2 Pectoral Fly/Day 1

Exercise Order

Day 1: Upper Body

1 Half Press Up
2 Pectoral Fly
3 Single Arm Row
4 Towel Pulldown
5 Shoulder Press
6 Lateral Raise
7 Bicep Curl
8 Bench Dips

Day 2: Lower Body

1 Sit Down Squat
2 Lunge
3 Glute Raise
4 Calf Raise
5 Half Bridge
6 Oblique Curl
7 Reverse Curl
8 Alternating Superman

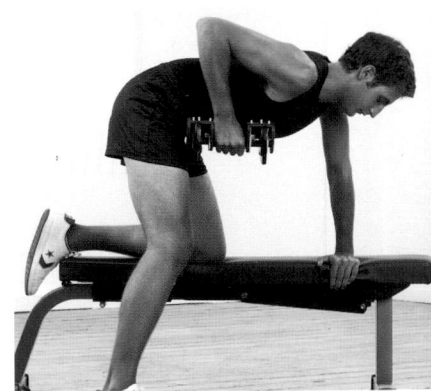

3 Single Arm Row/Day 1

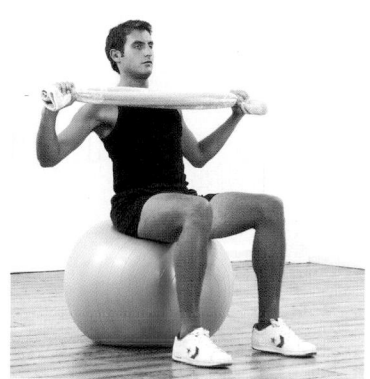

4 Towel Pulldown/Day 1

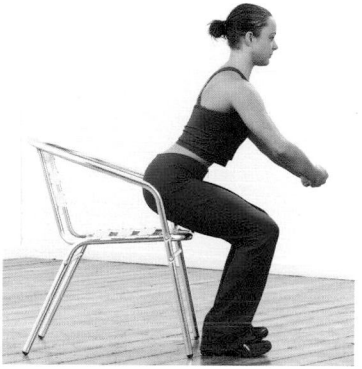

1 Sit Down Squat/Day 2

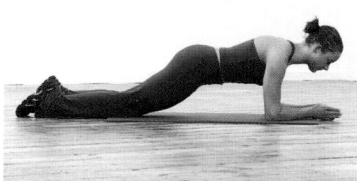

5 Half Bridge/Day 2

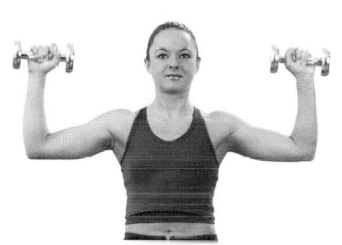

5 Shoulder Press/Day 1

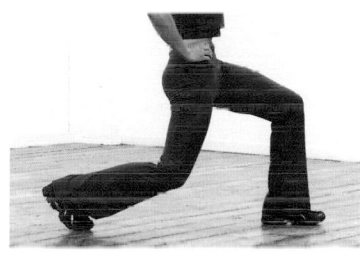

2 Lunge/Day 2

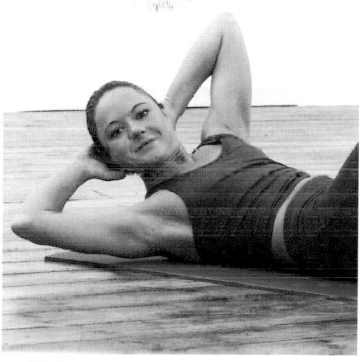

6 Oblique Curl/Day 2

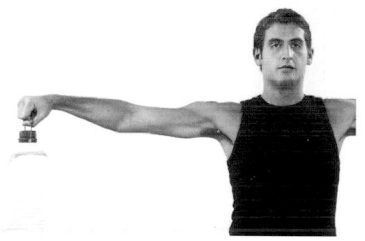

6 Lateral Raise/Day 1

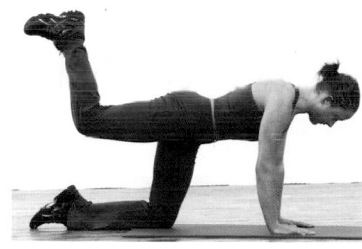

3 Glute Raise/Day 2

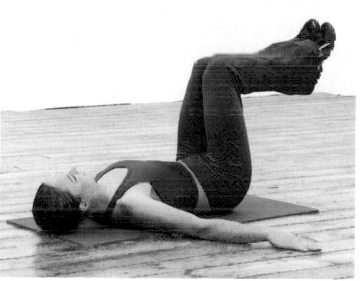

7 Reverse Curl/Day 2

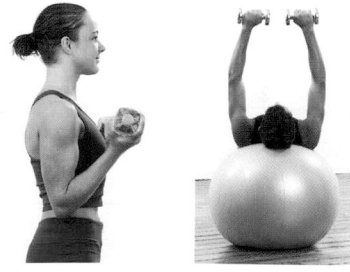

7 Bicep Curl/Day 1
8 Bench Press/Day 1

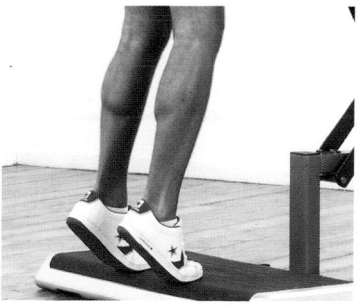

4 Calf Raise/Day 2

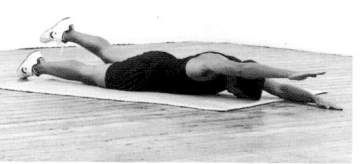

8 Alternating Superman/Day 2

Body Split—Advanced

one set to near muscular fatigue

Now you are really moving; and without a day off. You have come a long way from those early, tentative Half Press Ups.

Aims: To exercise a greater variety of muscles on separate days. One day to be spent concentrating on the upper body and one day on the lower body. While one set of muscles is working, the other muscles are resting, so that you can exercise on consecutive days.

Repetition Range: 10–15 repetitions. (Lifting two seconds. Lowering three+ seconds.)

Notes specific to workout: Still focus on the technique but aim to lift slightly heavier weights than you did in the base workout. You are only doing a single set so really focus on working hard. If you are getting to 15 repetitions and feel like you could do another three to five, increase the weight, where one is used, or if possible (and safe) increase range of movement.

Exercise Order

Day 1: Upper Body

1 Full Press Up
2 Decline Press Up
3 Pullover
4 Reverse Fly
5 Corkscrew Shoulder Press
6 Lateral Raise
7 Zottman Curl
8 Raised Dip

Day 2: Lower Body

1 Weighted Squats
2 Romanian Deadlift
3 Lunge
4 Calf Raise
5 Abdominal Crunch
6 Rotating Side Bridge
7 Heel Drops
8 Back Extension

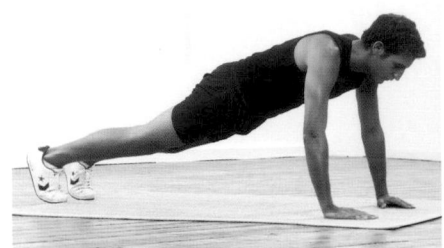

1 **Full Press Up/Day 1**

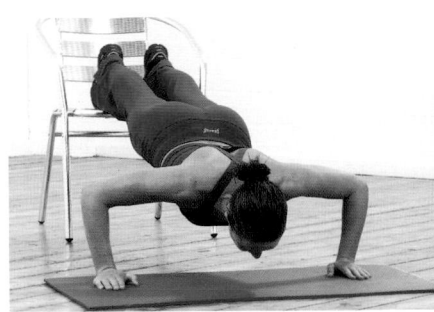

2 **Decline Press Up/Day 1**

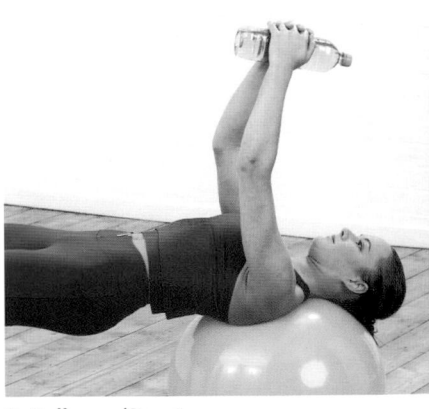

3 **Pullover/Day 1**

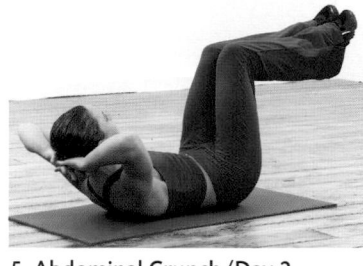

5 Abdominal Crunch/Day 2

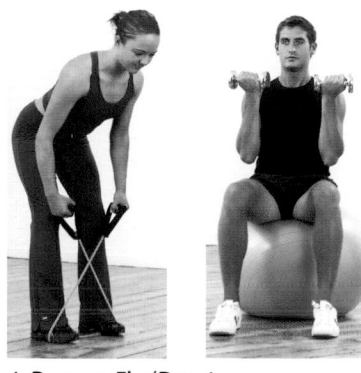

4 Reverse Fly/Day 1
5 Corkscrew Shoulder Press/Day 1

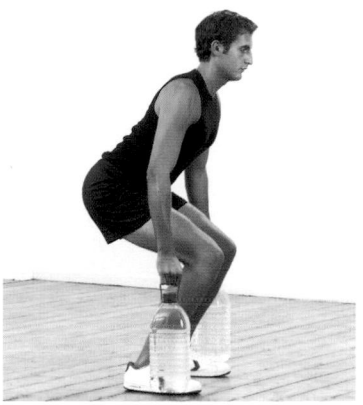

1 Weighted Squat/Day 2

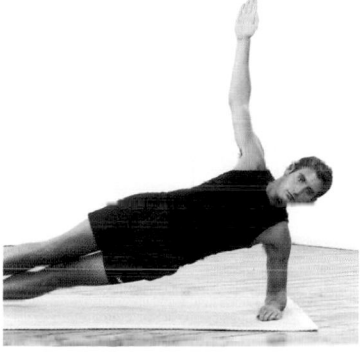

6 Rotating Side Bridge/Day 2

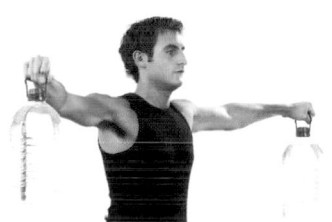

6 Lateral Raise/Day 1

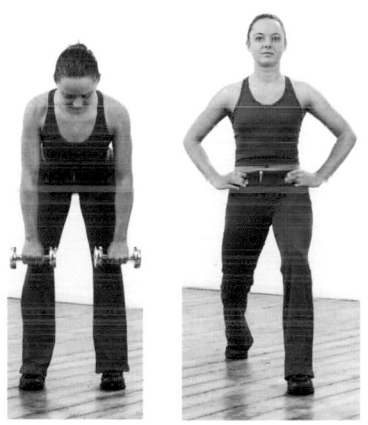

2 Romanian Deadlift/Day 2
3 Lunge/Day 2

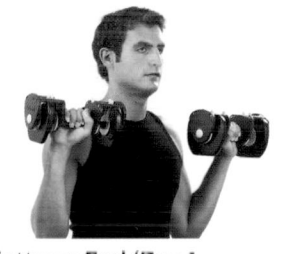

7 Zottman Curl/Day 1

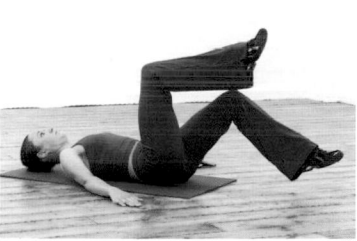

7 Heel Drops/Day 2

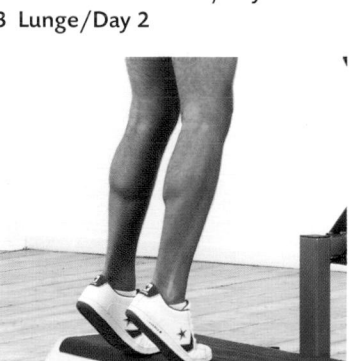

4 Calf Raise/Day 2

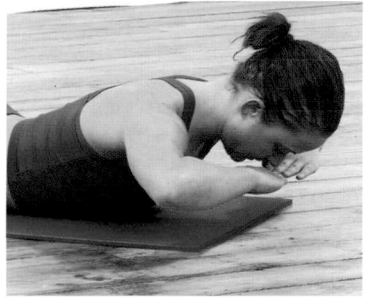

8 Back Extension/Day 2

8 Raised Dip/Day 1

Push/Pull–Beginner

one set to momentary muscular fatigue

Another body split, but this time with no obvious dividing line. Each limb and the trunk is split approximately, and opposing muscles work on consecutive days.

Aims: A variation on the previous two-day split routine but with similar aims. The repetition range is now going to come down slightly, so aim to bring the weights up. You are now mixing both lower body and upper body exercises on the same day. One day focuses on muscles responsible for pushing movement and one day on pulling movements. There are some gray areas such as shoulders, so if any muscles are still sore give them a little longer to rest.

Repetition Range: 8 to 12 repetitions. (Lifting two seconds. Lowering three+ seconds.)

Notes specific to workout: The workout is more taxing on your cardiovascular system owing to the variety of muscle groups that you are working. Your heart has to pump blood to all the muscles that are working. One minute it may be your legs, then another, your shoulders. Be aware that moving quickly from a lying position to a standing position may cause you to become light-headed. The first few times you do the workout, move from one exercise to the next slowly with a good rest (45 seconds to one minute) in between.

Exercise Order

Day 1: Push

1 Half Press Up
2 Sit Down Squat
3 Shoulder Press
4 Lunge
5 Bench Dip
6 Glute Raise
7 Supinated Tricep Extension
8 Alternating Superman

Day 2: Pull

1 Towel Pulldown
2 Single Arm Row
3 Shrugs
4 Bicep Curl
5 Half Bridge
6 Abdominal Curl
7 Reverse Curl
8 Oblique Curl

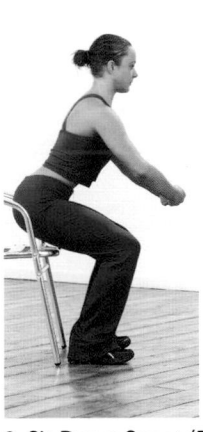
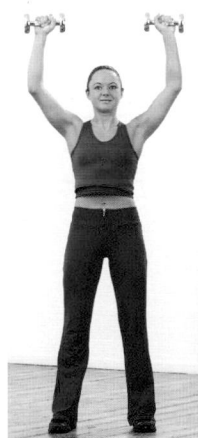

2 Sit Down Squat/Day 1
3 Shoulder Press/Day 1

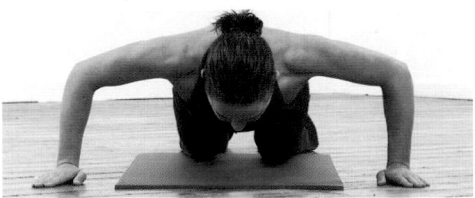

1 Half Press Up/Day 1

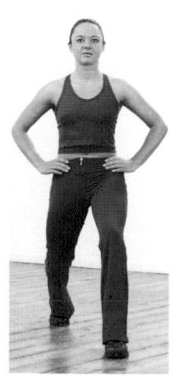

4 Lunge/Day 1
5 Bench Dip/Day 1

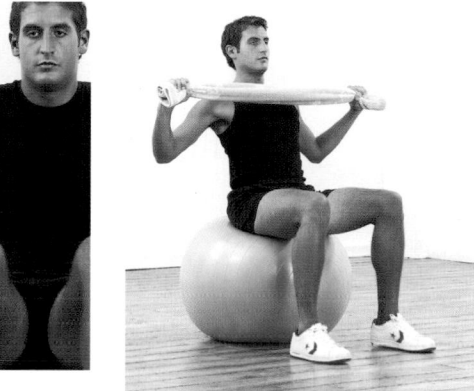

1 Towel Pulldown/Day 2

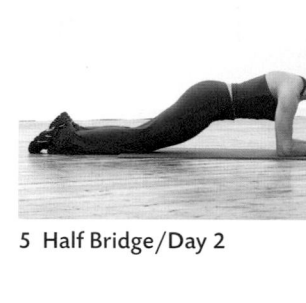

5 Half Bridge/Day 2

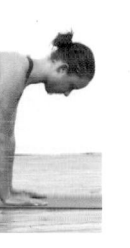

6 Glute Raise/Day 1

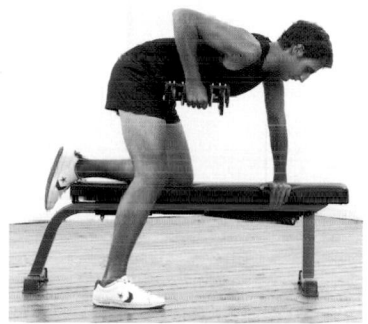

2 Single Arm Row/Day 2

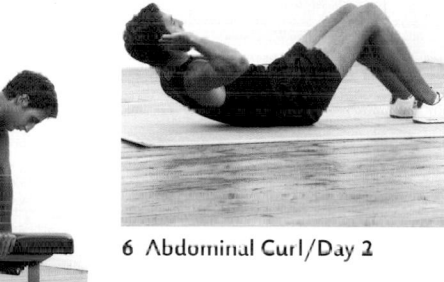

6 Abdominal Curl/Day 2

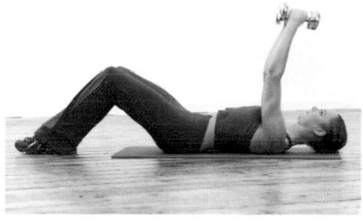

7 Supinated Tricep
Extension/Day 1

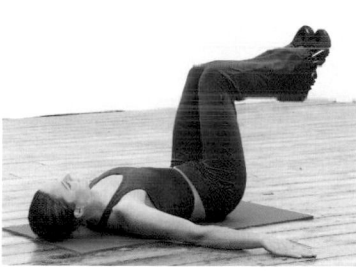

7 Reverse Curl/Day 2

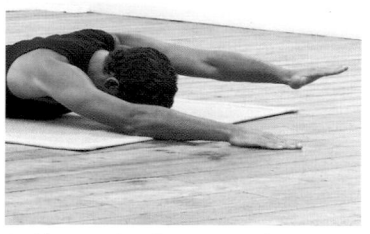

8 Alternating Superman/Day 1

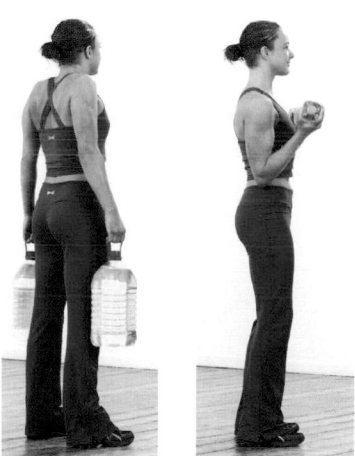

3 Shrugs/Day 2
4 Bicep Curl/Day 2

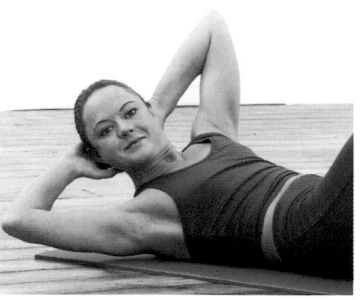

8 Oblique Curl/Day 2

Push/Pull—Advanced

one set to momentary muscular fatigue

Extension and flexion split once more—but this time it's serious. Push it away on Sunday and bring it back on Monday.

Aims: A variation on the previous two-day split routine but with similar aims. The repetition range is now going to come down slightly so bring the weights up. You are now mixing both lower body and upper body exercises on the same day. One day will focus on muscles responsible for pushing (extension) movement and one day on pulling (flexion) movements. Again, there are some gray areas such as shoulders so if any muscles are still sore give them a little longer to rest.

Repetition Range: 8–12 repetitions. (Lifting two seconds. Lowering three+ seconds.)

Notes specific to workout: The workout will be more taxing on your cardiovascular system owing to the variety of muscle groups that you are using. Your heart has to pump blood to all the muscles that are working: one minute your legs, another, your shoulders. Be aware that moving quickly from a lying to a standing position may cause you to become light headed. The first few times you do the workout, move from one exercise to the next with a good rest (45 seconds to one minute) in between.

Exercise Order

Day 1: Push

1 Full/3 Point Press Up
2 Weighted Squat
3 Decline Press Up
4 Plié Squat
5 Corkscrew Shoulder Press
6 Raised Dip
7 Calf Raise
8 Back Extension

Day 2: Pull

1 Pullover
2 Romanian Deadlift
3 Bent Over Row
4 Upright Row
5 Bicep Curl
6 Zottman Curl
7 Full Crunch
8 Heel Drops

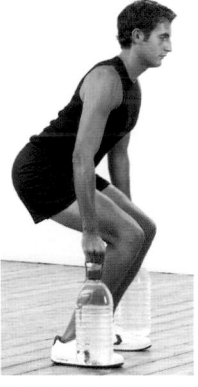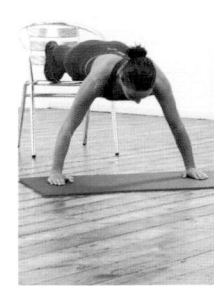

2 Weighted Squat/Day 1
3 Decline Press Up/Day 1

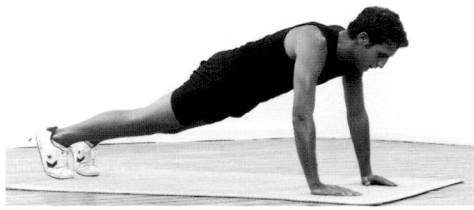

1 Full or 3 Point Press Up/Day 1

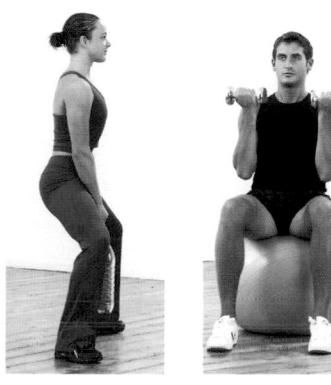

4 Plié Squat/Day 1
5 Corkscrew Shoulder Press/Day 1

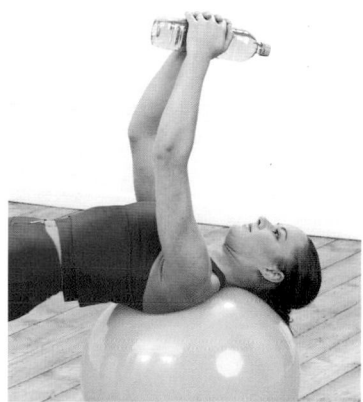

1 Pullover/Day 2

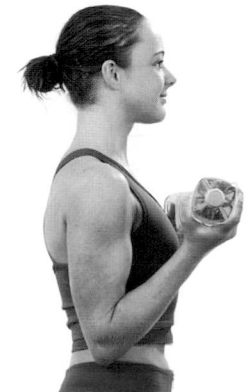

5 Bicep Curl/Day 2

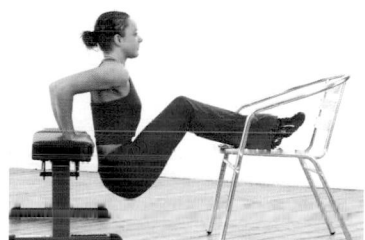

6 Raised Dip/Day 1

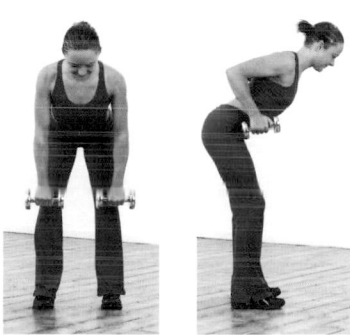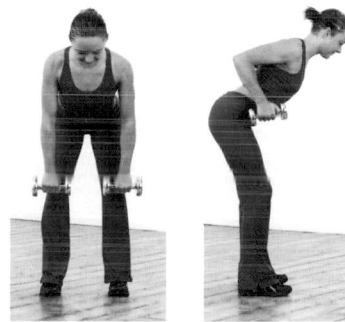

2 Romanian Deadlift/Day 2
3 Bent Over Row/Day 2

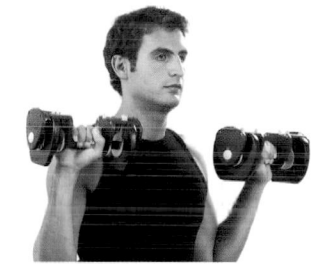

6 Zottman Curl/Day 2

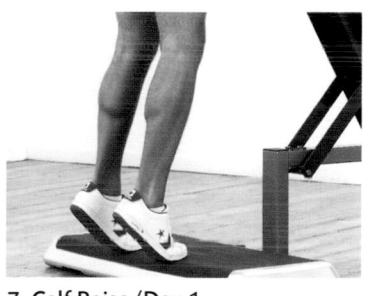

7 Calf Raise/Day 1

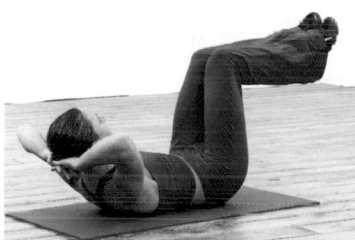

7 Full Crunch/Day 2

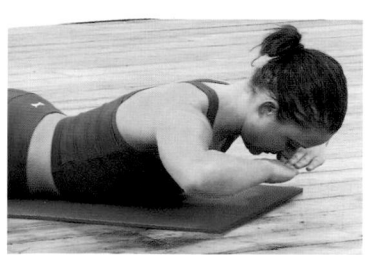

8 Back Extension/Day 1

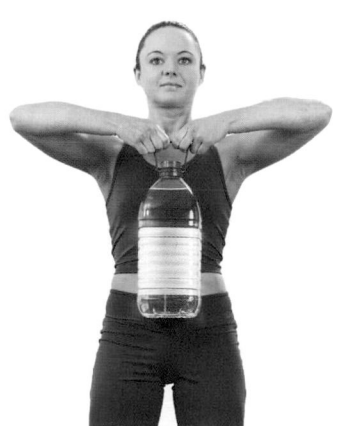

4 Upright Row/Day 2

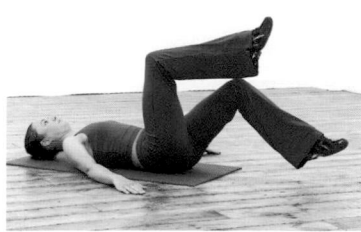

8 Heel Drops/Day 2

Superset–Beginners

two to three circuits

Not repetitions, but time as the limiting factor; burn off that over-indulgent lunch by going for the full minute.

Aims: To improve muscular endurance and burn as many calories as possible. The workout consists of large compound movements and is time- rather than repetition-based.

Repetition Range: As many repetitions under control in one minute.

Notes specific to workout: Complete one minute on the exercise and then move on to the next. Try to keep rest times to a minimum. When you have completed all exercises, rest and repeat the circuit again using slightly heavier weights. Continue this cycle two to three times.

Exercise Order

1 Half Press Ups
2 Single Arm Row
3 Lunge (switch sides after 30 seconds)
4 Shoulder Press
5 Abdominal Curl
6 Alternating Superman

Complete two to three minutes of step-ups on stairs or low bench/box at a gentle pace. Rest and repeat circuit once or twice more.

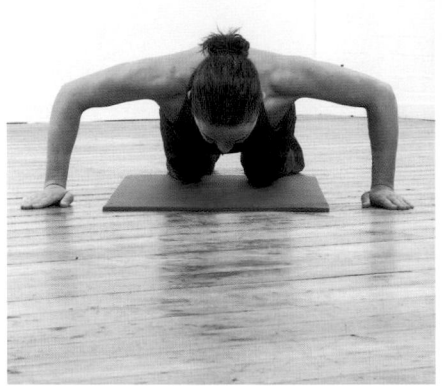

1 **Half Press Ups**

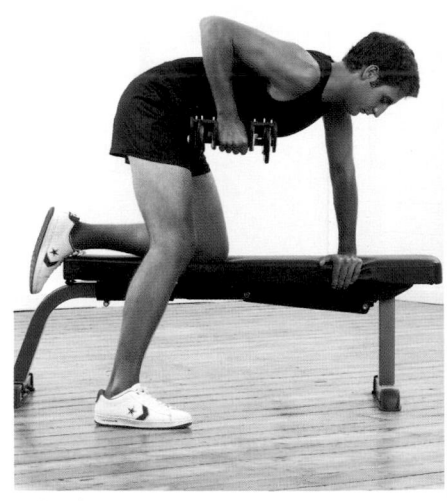

2 **Single Arm Row**

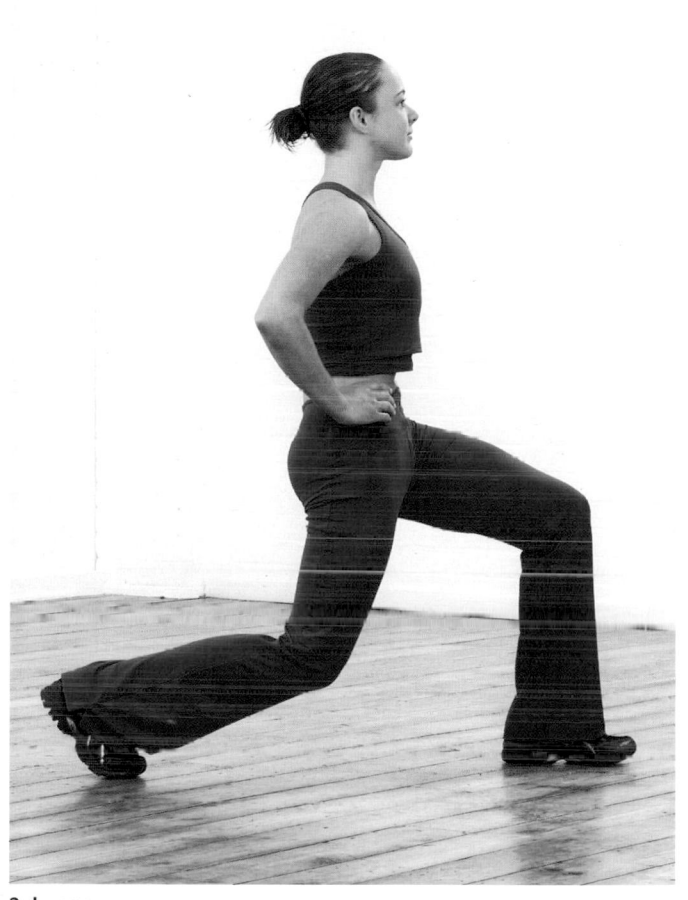

3 Lunge

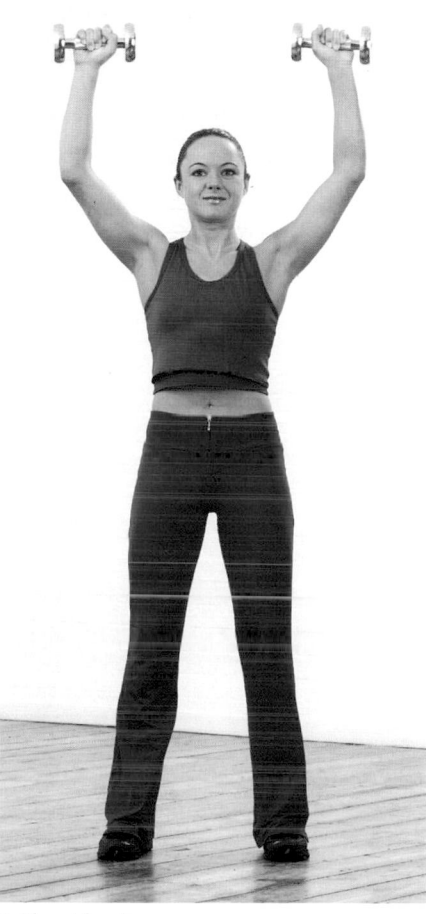

4 Shoulder Press

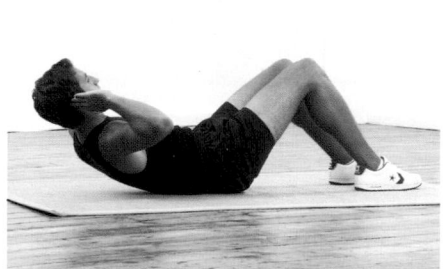

5 Abdominal Curl

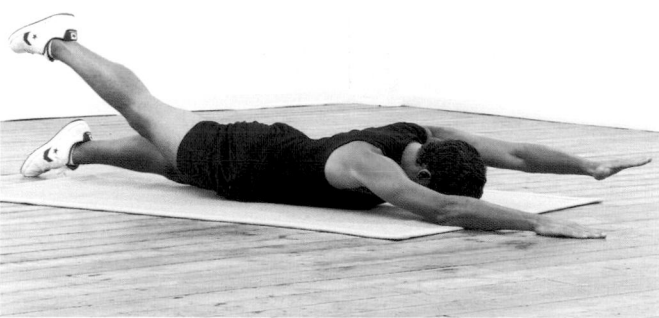

6 Alternating Superman

Superset—Advanced

two to three circuits

Do not cheat yourself by working too slowly, but at the same time, do not lose technique for the sake of a few more repetitions.

Aims: To improve muscular endurance and burn as many calories as possible. The workout consists of large, compound movements and is time- rather than repetition-based.

Repetition Range: As many repetitions as you can, under control, in one minute.

Notes specific to workout: Complete one minute on the exercise and then move on to the next. Try to keep rest times to a minimum. When you have completed all exercises rest and repeat the circuit again using slightly heavier weights. Continue this cycle two to three times.

Exercise Order

1 Decline Press Ups
2 Bent Over Row
3 Power Squats
4 Shoulder Push Press
5 Knuckled Close Grip Press Up
6 Abdominal Crunch

Complete two to three minutes of step-ups on stairs or low bench/box at a gentle pace. Rest and repeat circuit once or twice more.

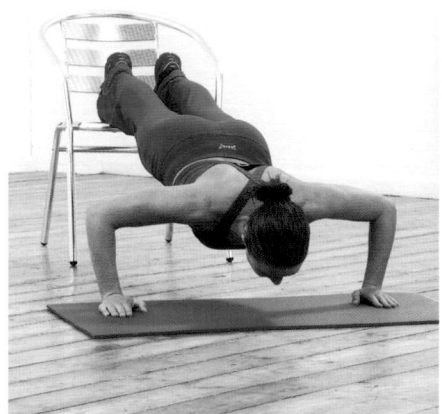

1 **Decline Press Ups**

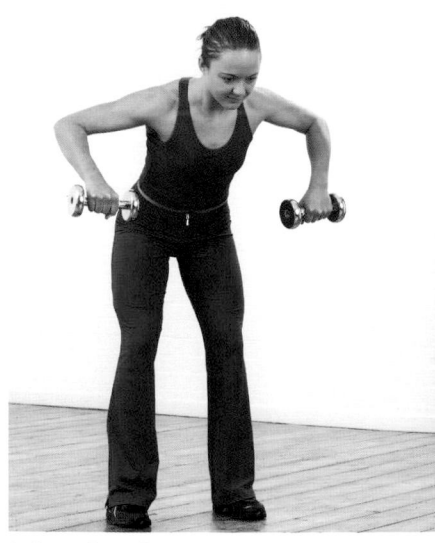

2 **Bent Over Row**

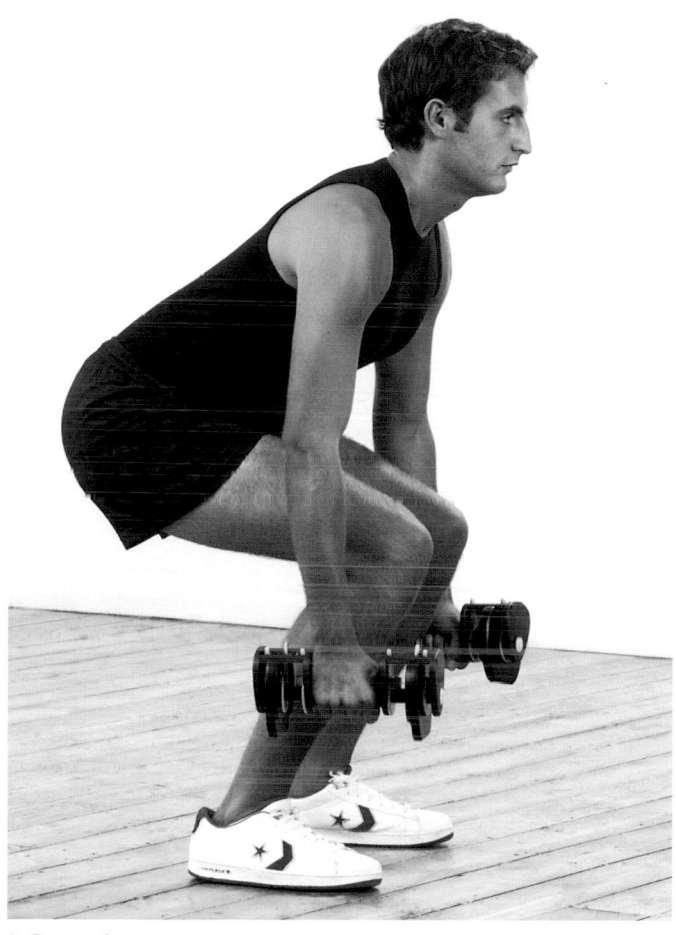

3 Power Squat

4 Shoulder Press

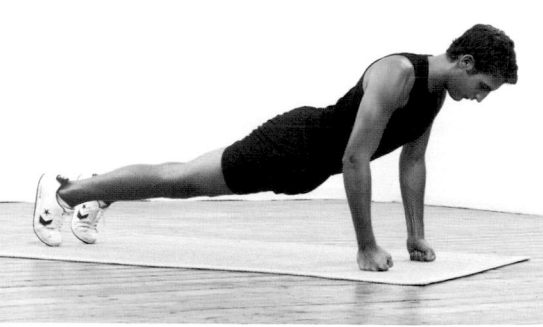

5 Knuckled Close Grip Press Up

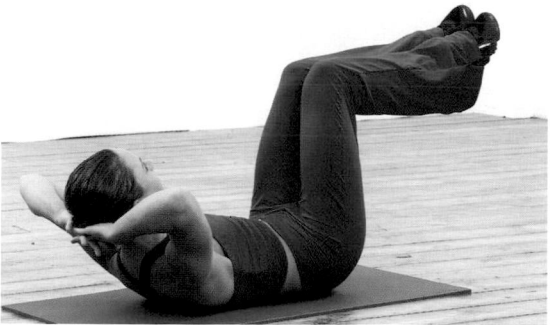

6 Abdominal Crunch

Strength–Beginners

three sets (final set to muscular fatigue)

The third set is the key. The first two are to prepare the muscles to reach closer to the point of fatigue so that the heavier weights can really challenge them.

Aims: To increase the maximum weight that you can lift. You will become stronger lifting weights overall—that is, for whatever activity you undertake—but this is a workout that you can use specifically to focus on being able to lift heavier weights. The exercise demands large compound movements and should only be done two to three times a week to give the body adequate recovery time.

Repetition Range: 6–8 repetitions.

Notes specific to workout: The initial set should be light with each following set becoming heavier. This is to prepare your body for the final set, which should be to muscular fatigue. Rest for approximately 30 seconds to one minute between sets. Note that when lifting heavy weights it is always important to use good technique and preferable to have someone there to spot you (cover the weight for you).

Exercise Order

1 Bench Press
2 Sit Down Squat (Use weights in hands or progress to Weighted Squat)
3 Shoulder Press
4 Single Arm Row

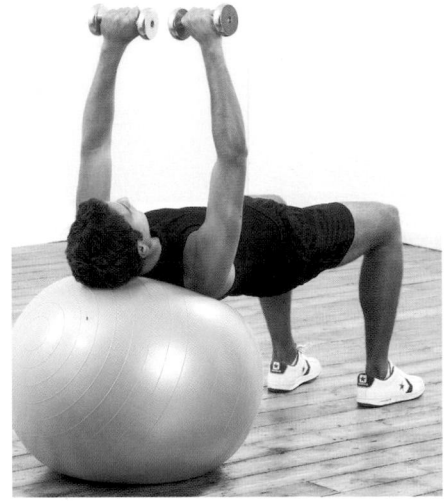

1 Bench Press

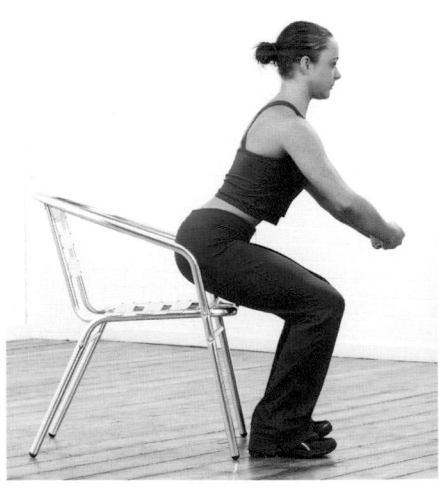

2 Sit Down Squat

3 Single Arm Row

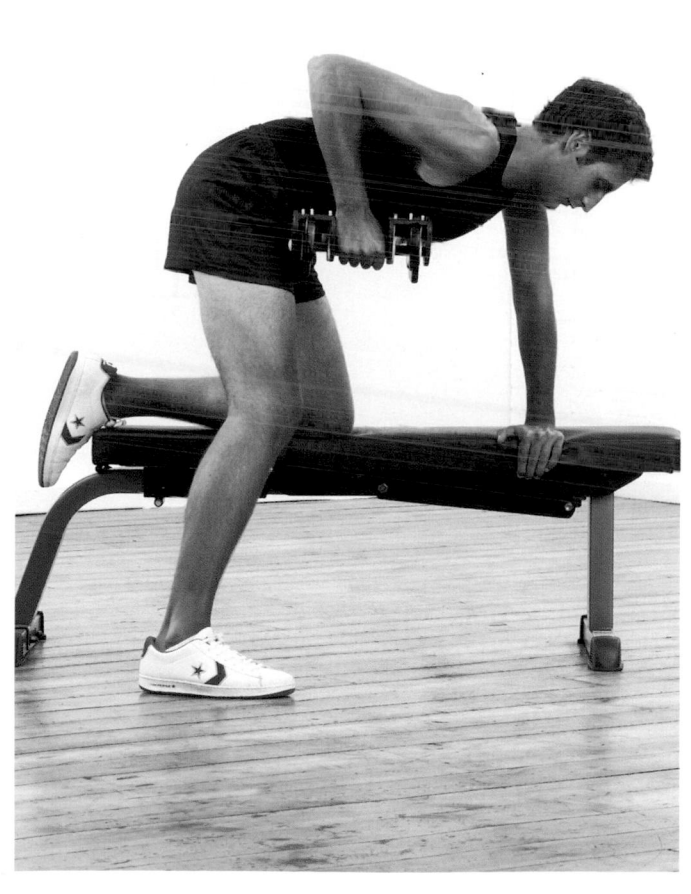

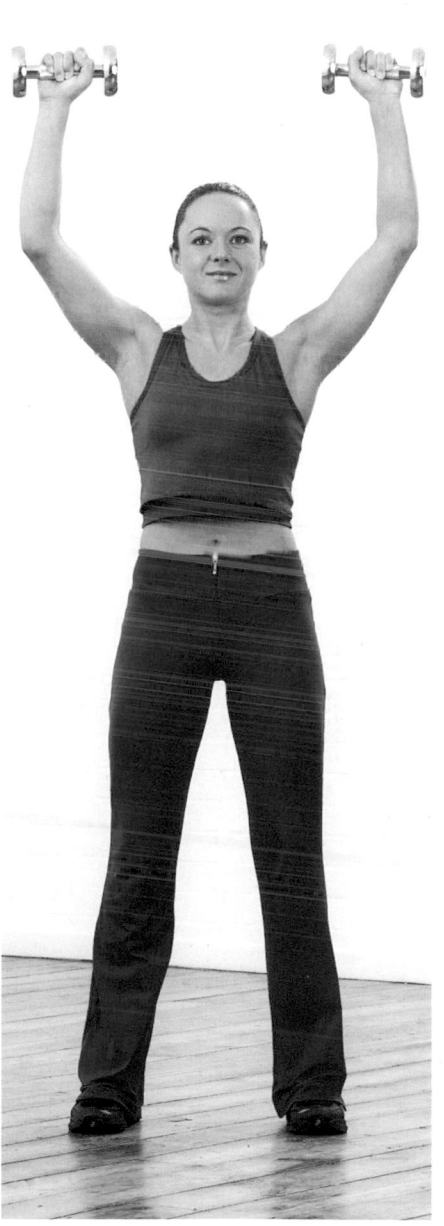

4 Shoulder Press

Strength–Advanced

sets specific to exercise

The Clean and Press works all the major muscle groups, which is why some consider it to be the premier event of competitive weightlifting.

Aims: To increase the maximum weight that you can lift. You will become stronger lifting weights overall—that is, for whatever activity you undertake—but this is a workout that you can use specifically to focus on being able to lift heavier weights. The workout focuses on the Clean and Press exercise. You will be gradually building up the exercise by focussing on each element of the lift individually.

Repetition Range: 6–8 repetitions.

Notes specific to workout: The Clean and Press is a large movement so you need plenty of space. Stretch your hands over your head before you begin to make sure that you will not hit the ceiling when you are holding the weights. The initial set should be light, with each following set becoming heavier. On the first three of the following exercises do not go to muscular fatigue.

Exercise Order

1 Deadlift (2 sets)
2 Clean (2 sets)
3 Shoulder Push Press (2 sets)
4 Clean and Press (3 sets: Sets 1 and 2 focus on correct technique with lighter weights. Set 3 is the working set).

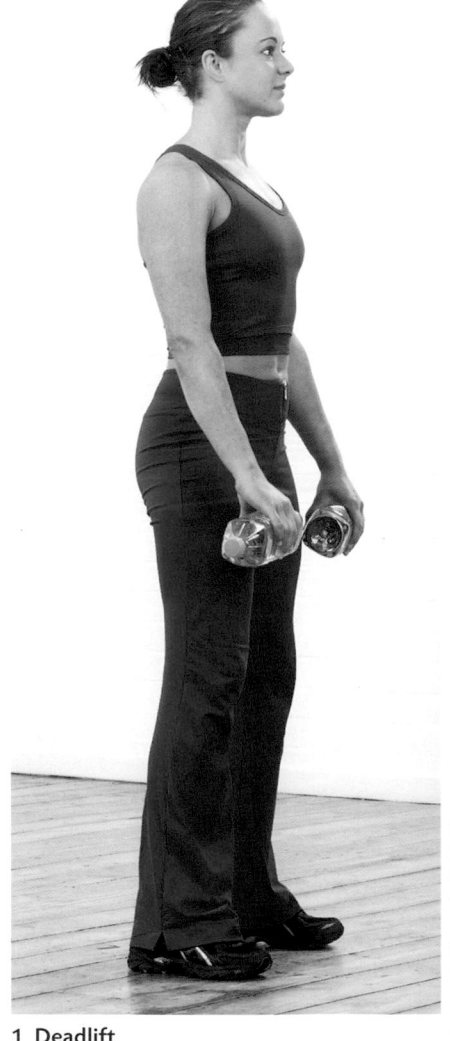

1 Deadlift

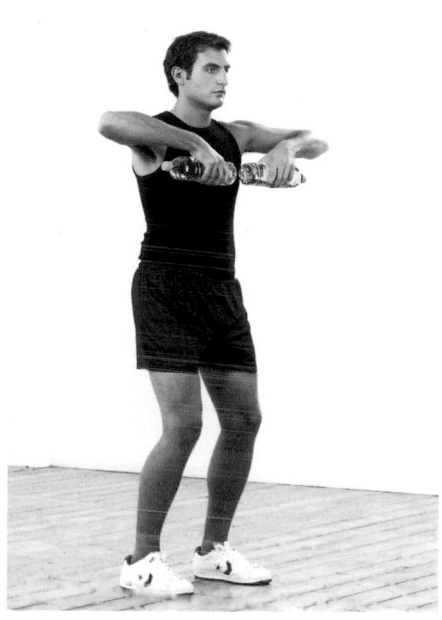

2 Clean

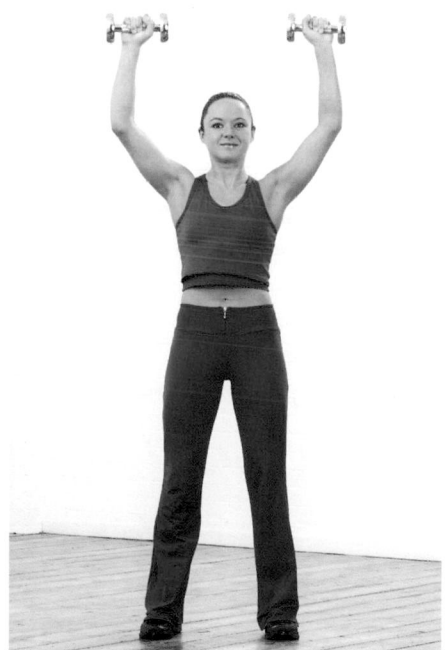

3 Shoulder Press

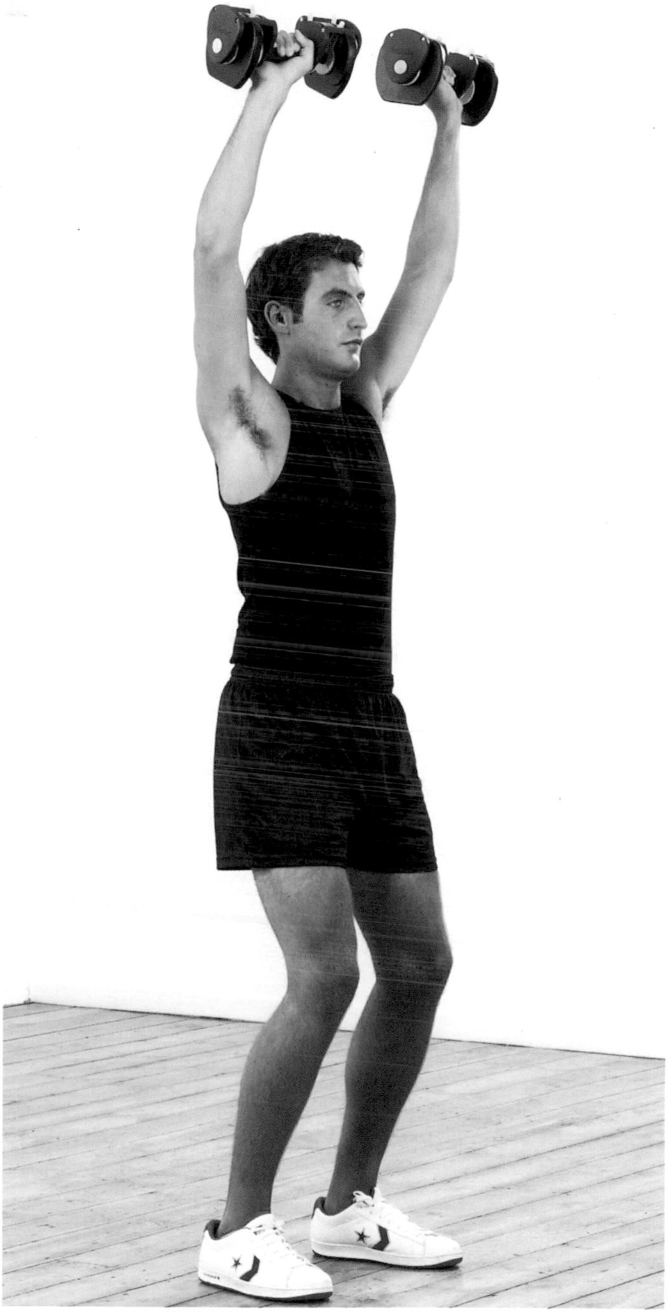

4 Clean and Press

Pre-Fatigue–Beginner
one set to momentary muscle fatigue

Working the muscles twice, hopefully for more than double the effect; first in isolation, then as part of a compound exercise.

Aims: To continue to challenge the muscles, with additional weight to lift as the limiting factor. Because of the nature of these exercises you will be getting stronger, so weights that were once challenging to lift may now be feeling comfortable. Therefore this workout is designed to make the muscles work hard individually; then, when performing an exercise where they work with others, the muscles will already be tired, thus making the exercise more challenging.

Repetition Range: 8–12 repetitions. (Lifting two seconds. Lowering three seconds.)

Notes specific to workout: The exercises are in pairs. One pre-fatigue isolation exercise is followed by a compound exercise. Keep rest times to a minimum between the first and second exercises in each pair.

Exercise Order

1 Pectoral Fly
2 Bench Press
3 Glute Raise
4 Lunge
5 Shrug
6 Single Arm Row
7 Lateral Raise
8 Shoulder Press
9 Half Bridge
10 Alternating Superman

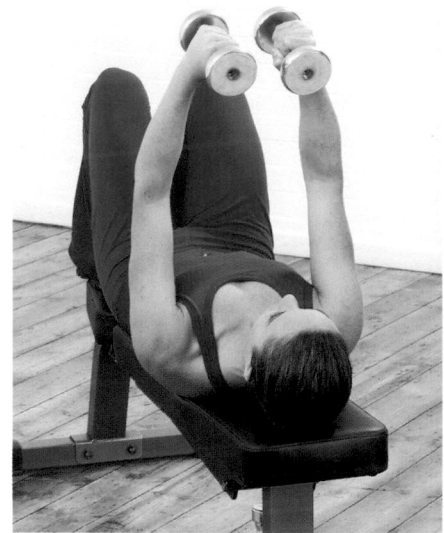

1 Pectoral Fly

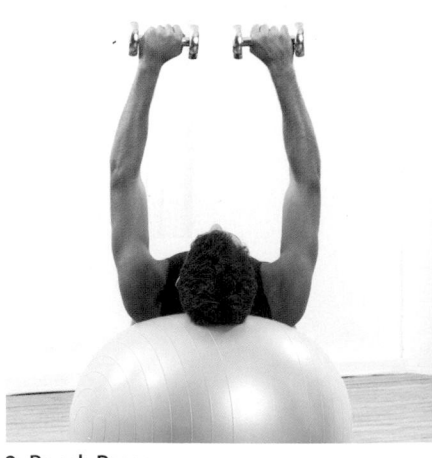

2 Bench Press

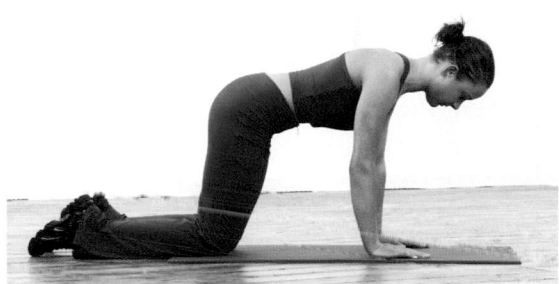

3 Glute Raise

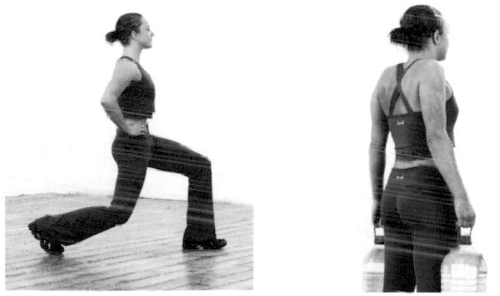

4 Lunge 5 Shrug

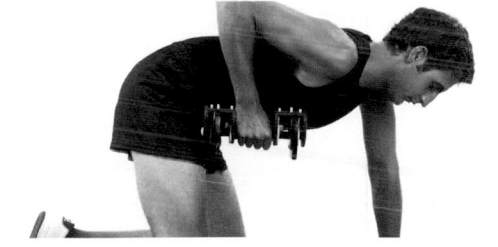

6 Single Arm Row

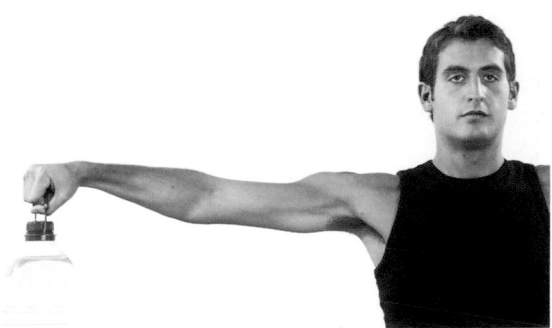

7 Lateral Raise

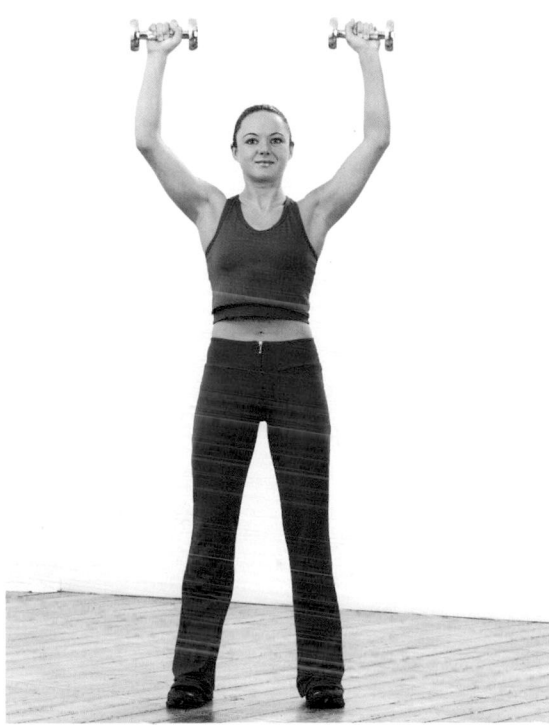

8 Shoulder Press

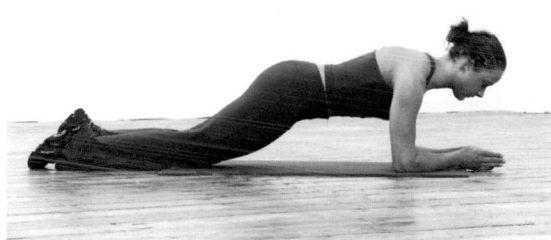

9 Half Bridge

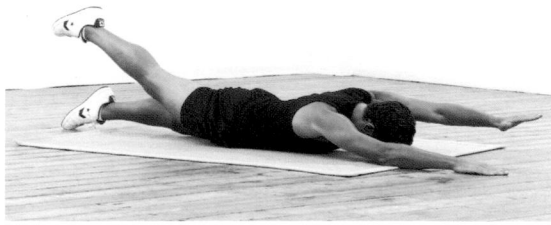

10 Alternating Superman

Pre-Fatigue–Advanced

one set to momentary muscular fatigue

Just a quick glance at the photographs reveals the thinking behind this workout: the exercises are quite obviously in pairs.

Aims: To continue to challenge the muscles, with additional weight to lift as the limiting factor. Because of the nature of these exercises you will be getting stronger, so weights that were once challenging to lift may now be feeling comfortable. Therefore this workout is designed to make the muscles work hard individually; then, when performing an exercise where they work with others, the muscles will already be tired, thus making the exercise more challenging. This workout can also be used specifically to challenge different muscles under fatigue for sport-related training.

Repetition Range: 8–12 repetitions. (Lifting two seconds. Lowering three seconds.)

Notes specific to workout: The exercises are in pairs. One pre-fatigue isolation exercise is followed by a compound exercise Keep rest times to a minimum between the first and second exercises in each pair.

Exercise Order

1 Reverse Fly
2 Bent Over Row
3 Upright Row
4 Shoulder Press
5 Weighted Squat
6 Romanian Deadlift
7 Pectoral Fly
8 Decline Press Up
9 Full Bridge
10 Knuckled Close Grip Press Up

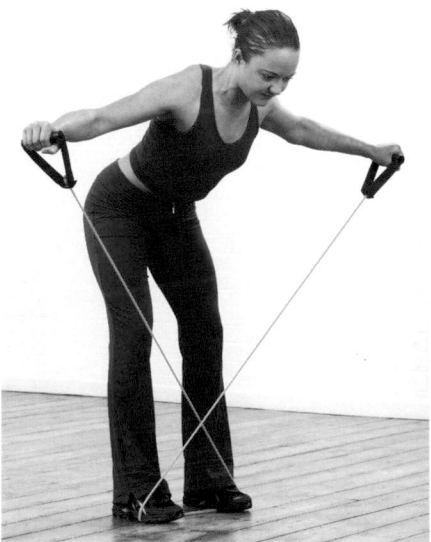

1 Reverse Fly

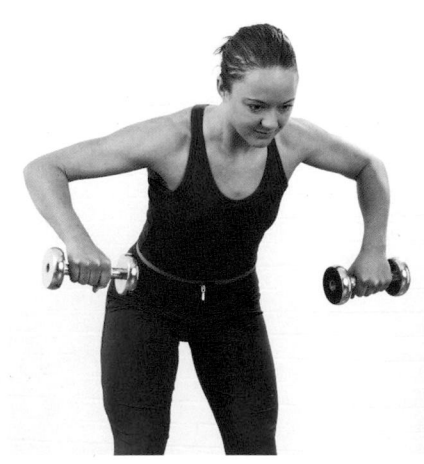

2 Bent Over Row

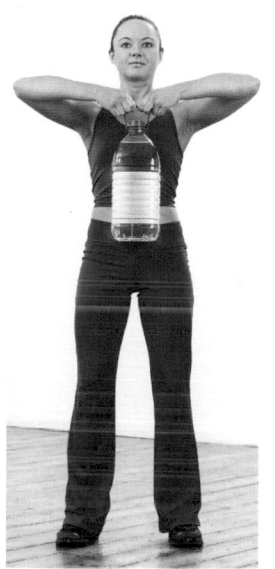

3 Upright Row

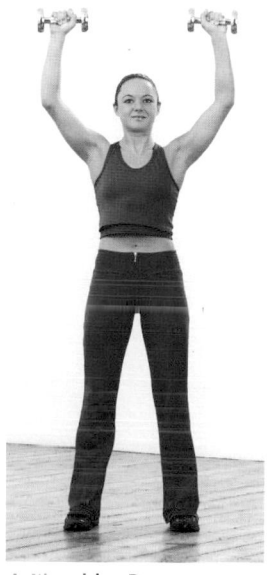

4 Shoulder Press

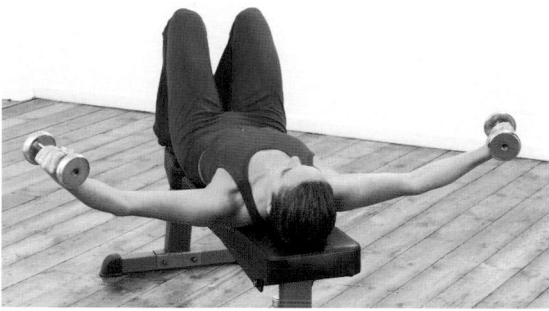

7 Pectoral Fly

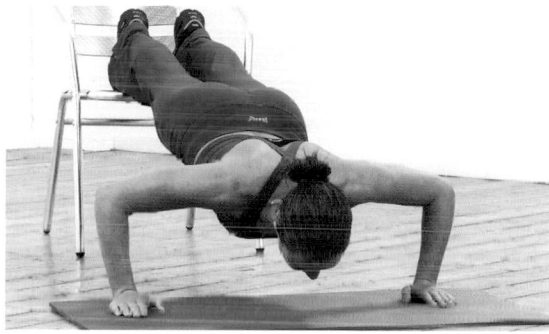

8 Decline Press Up

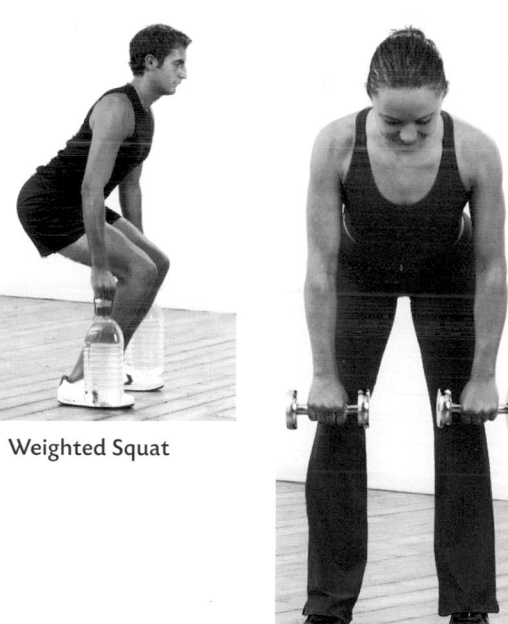

5 Weighted Squat

6 Romanian Deadlift

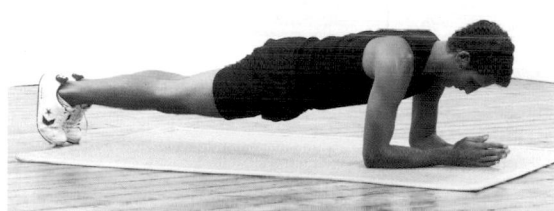

9 Full Bridge

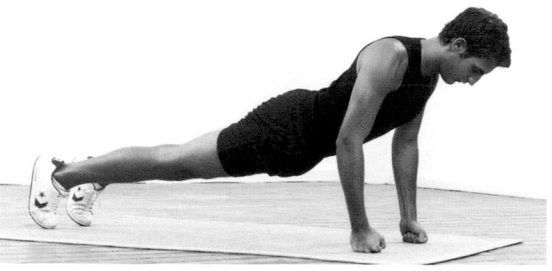

10 Knuckled Close Grip Press Up

More Challenging

stability ball pike and press

Area Worked: Upper thigh, stomach, chest, back of the arms, and front of shoulders.
Name of Muscles: Hip Flexor, Abdominals, Pectoralis, Triceps, and Anterior Deltoid.

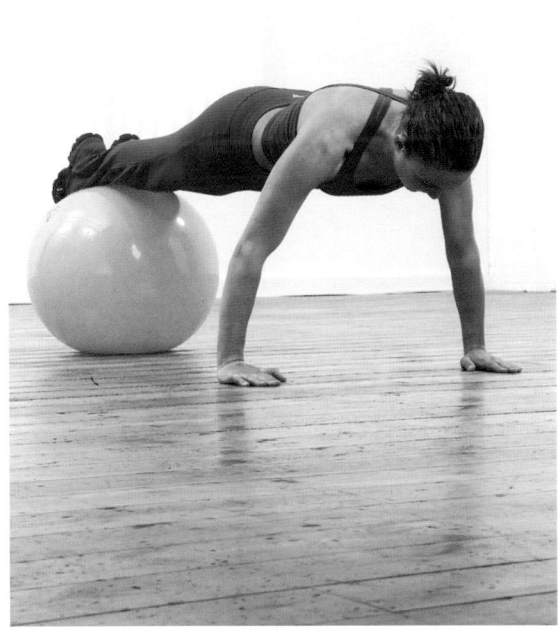 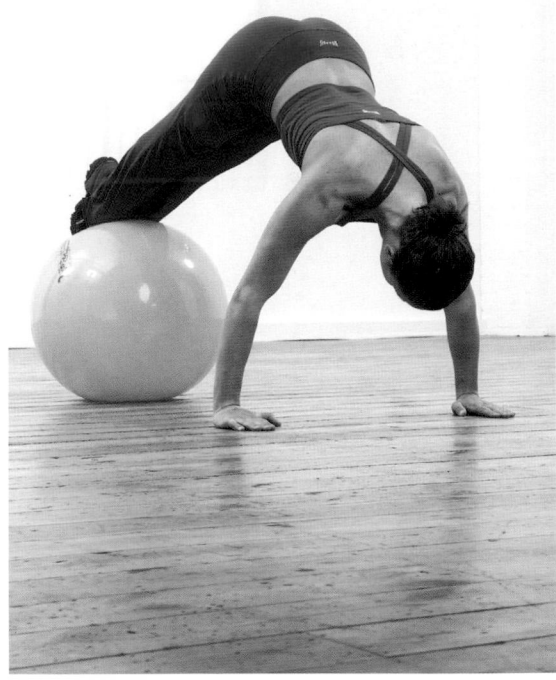

1 Position yourself over a stability ball so that you are supporting yourself with your hands on the floor and your shins on the ball.

2 Push your hips in to the air and pull the ball in underneath you. This is the Pike.

Hints & Tips

- To work the triceps more, use a narrow grip press up as in the Close Grip Knuckled Press Up. This is usually harder than a standard press up.

Technique

The following exercises are for those who have mastered all that has gone before— and a reminder that there is always some new way to enliven your resistance workouts to keep boredom at bay.

- Keep your abdominal muscles braced throughout the exercise. Be careful that you do not allow your hips to drop or your back to arch. You should have a straight line through your body from shoulder to hip.

- Before starting the Pike section, pull your abdominal muscles in and push your hips up. Use your abs to pull the ball in. Keep the knees soft and start slowly to make the muscles work harder and keep momentum to a minimum.

- When you are about to start the press, do a quick mental body check. Think about where your upper body is in relation to your hands. Your chest should be directly over your hands with your elbows soft. Your back should be straight, without arching, and your knees should be soft.

- Lower slowly and try not to push your head forward. Ideally, your chest should come to within a couple of inches of the floor while maintaining good posture; but if you can't get that far, work through a range of movement that is comfortable and increase as you become stronger.

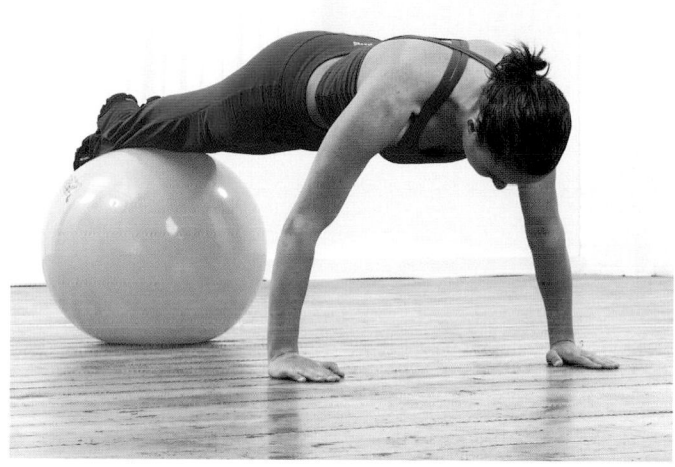

3 Roll the ball slowly back out to the start position.

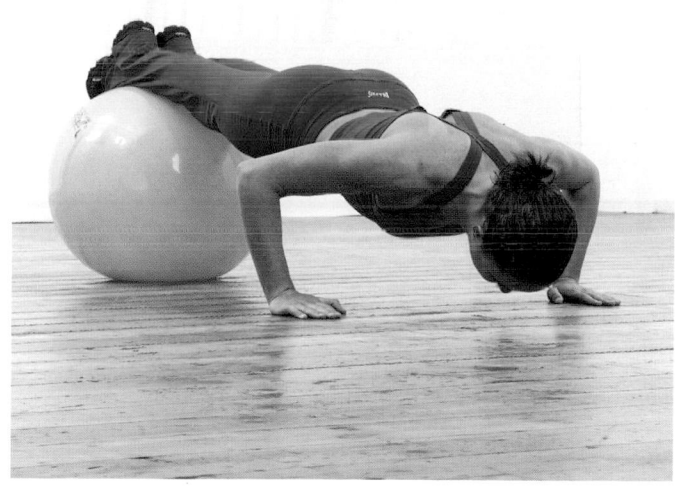

4 Bend your elbows and lower your chest toward the floor, then push to straighten your arms and return to the start position. This is the Press; you have completed one repetition.

More Challenging

stability ball lateral crunch

Area Worked: Side of stomach.
Name of Muscles: Obliques.

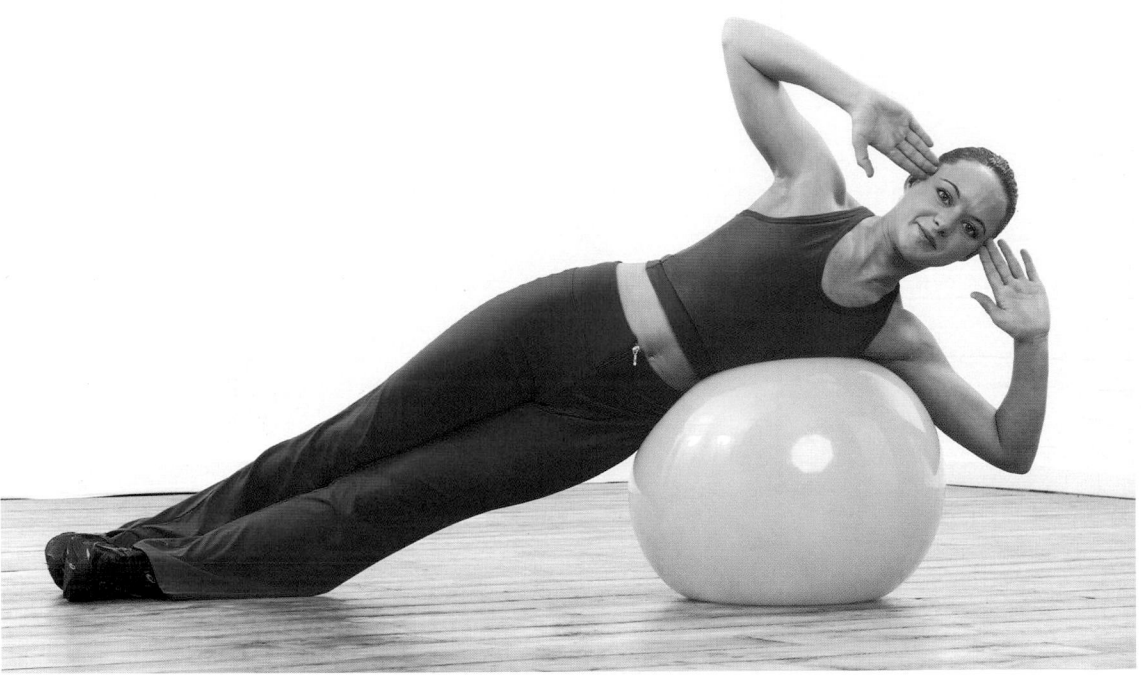

1 Lay on your side over the stability ball with your feet split.

Hints & Tips

- Vary the arm position to make the exercise easier or harder. Placing your hands across your chest is the easiest.
- Finger tips at the temples is the "middle option" and is the one most often used.
- Extending your arms up and over your head is the hardest. The straighter they go the harder it becomes.

Technique

- Balance is a major issue in this exercise. The farther apart you split your feet, the more stable you become. Which leg you move forward and which leg you place at the back is up to you. Find which way works best for you. Avoid shiny surfaces.

- Your initial position on the ball also determines how difficult the exercise is. Try to lie directly in the middle of the ball. You should place your hip approximately two-thirds of the way up the ball. This should mean you are supported through your hip and your rib cage.

- The range of movement is relatively small. Move as if you were trying to pull your shoulder up over your hip and focus on keeping your body straight. Twisting the body will only move the emphasis onto other muscles.

- Always look straight ahead and try not to tilt the head in the direction that you are lifting.

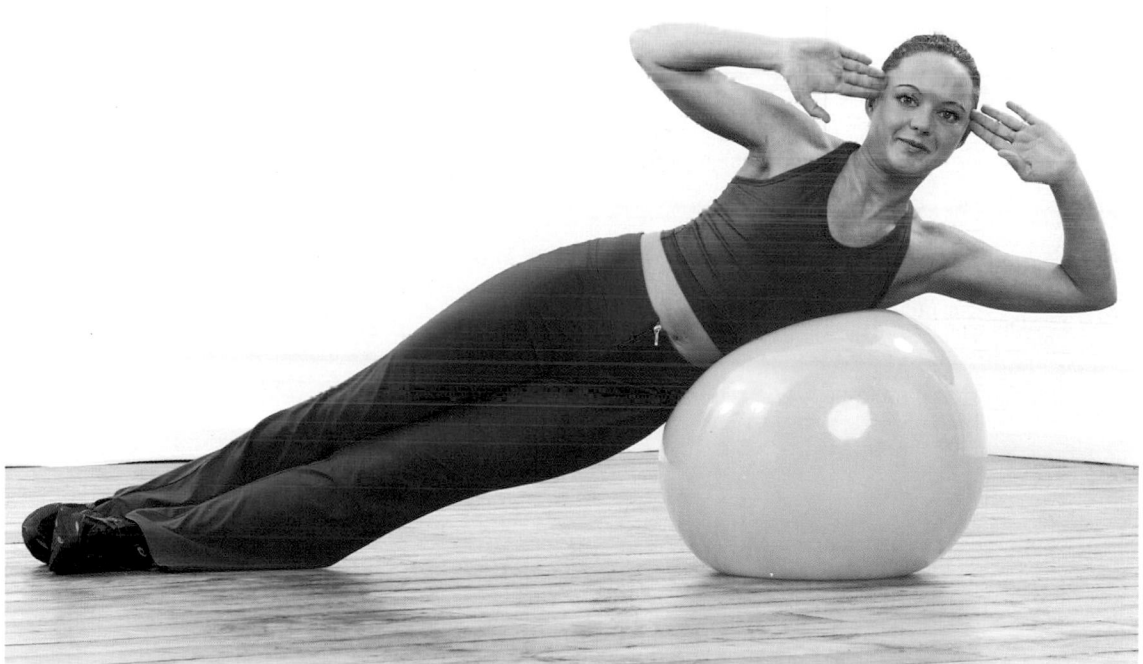

2 Keeping the body straight (not leaning backward or forward), lift up, bringing your ribs off the ball. Slowly lower back down and repeat.

More Challenging

v-sit twist

Area Worked: Stomach.
Name of Muscles: Obliques and Transverse Abdominus.

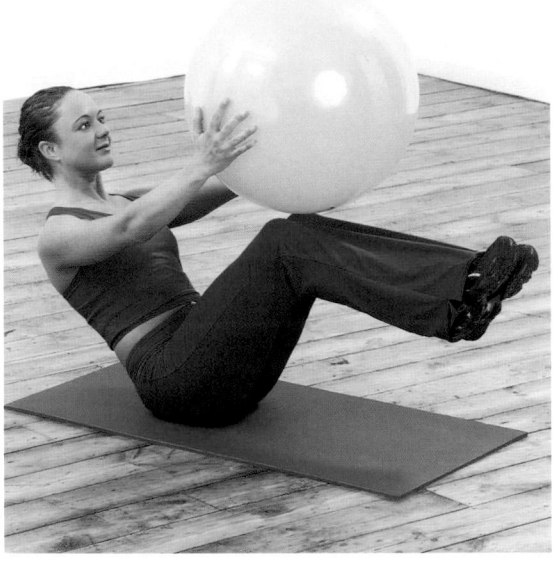
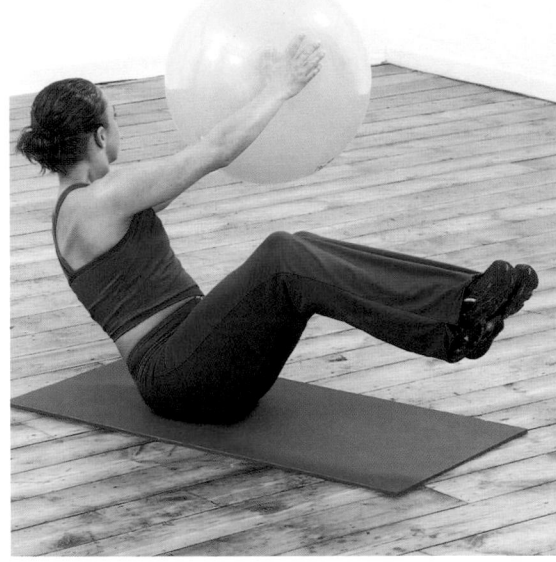

1 Sit on the floor holding a small stability ball, medicine ball, or other object that can be held comfortably. Tip back slightly and lift the feet from the floor so that you are balanced with your butt on the floor.

2 Holding the object in your hands at arm's length, rotate the upper body round. Return back to the center and repeat in the opposite direction.

Hints & Tips

- The heavier the object the harder the exercise becomes, but be aware that it is the muscles in the front of your shoulders that have to bear the weight. These tend to fatigue before your abs, so select a challenging but manageable weight.

Technique

- Posture is very important. Hold yourself high. Lift the chest, pull the shoulders back, and keep the abdominals tight. It requires a lot of strength to maintain this position. Be careful that your lower back does not round. If it does, it means your abdominal muscles have done as much as they can.

- The straighter you make your legs, the harder the exercise becomes. Start with the knees bent and as you become stronger, straighten them out.

- Keep the arms straight out in front, level with the chest. As you rotate, the arms should always be level and central to the chest. Keep your eyes on the ball at all times as you twist.

- Keep the movement slow. You are only rotating your shoulders and torso. Your hips shouldn't move during the movement. Rotate as far as you can comfortably go before switching direction.

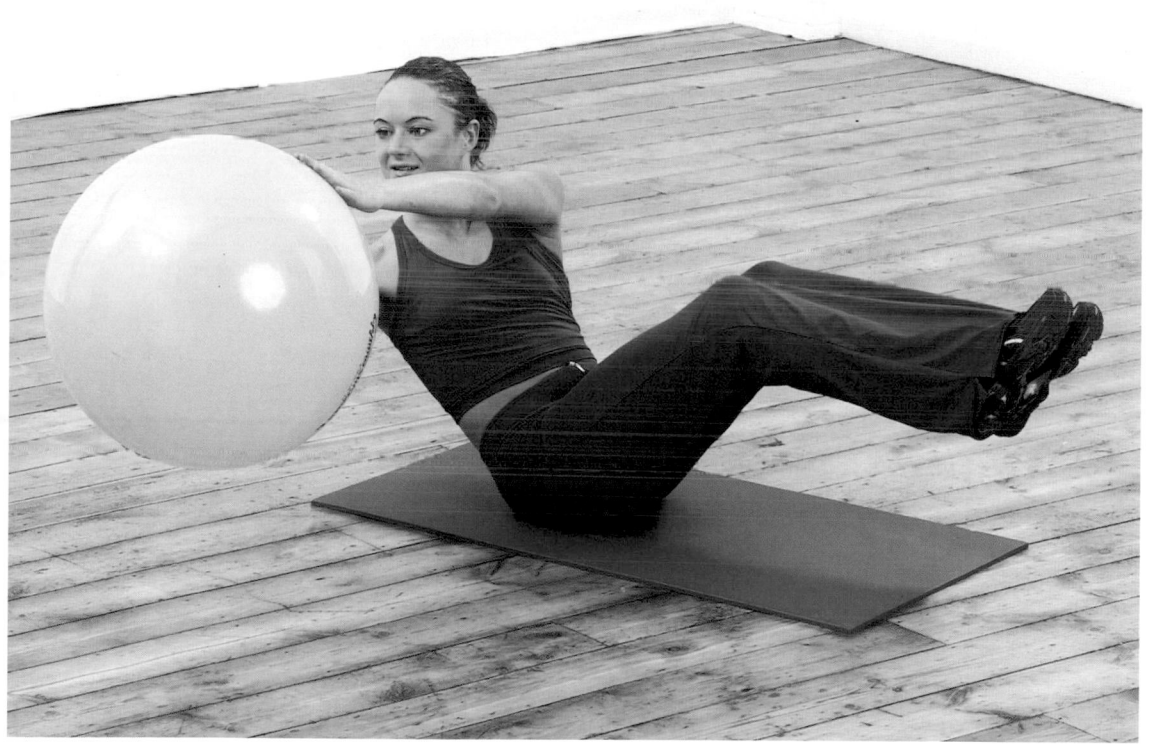

3 Alternate the sides for the desired number of repetitions.

More Challenging

stability ball iso leg curl

Area Worked: Back of thighs, butt, and lower back.
Name of Muscles: Hamstrings and Gluteals.

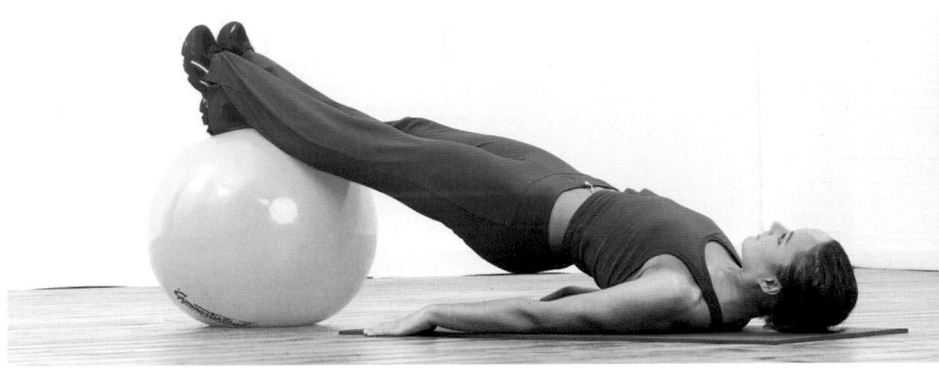

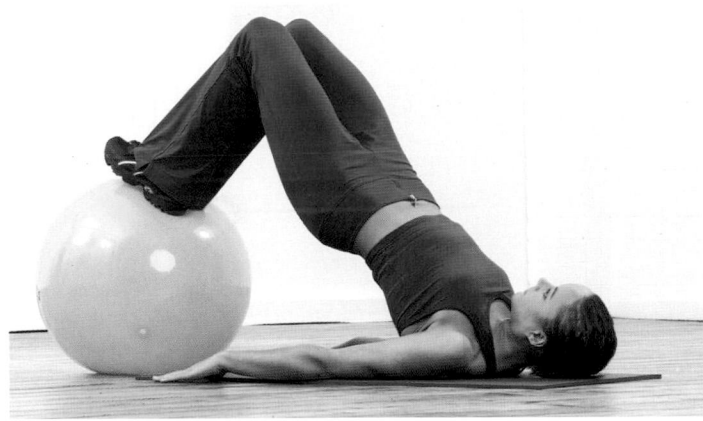

1 Lie on your back on the floor with your calves and ankles resting on a stability ball. Place your arms on the floor by your sides.

2 Push against the ball with your legs and raise your hips from the floor. Pull the ball underneath you and hold in this position.

Hints & Tips

• When you feel confident with the exercise, try taking your hands from the floor. This will mean that you will have to work much harder to maintain your balance.

Technique

- When lifting your hips from the floor try to keep the body in a straight line from your feet to your shoulders.

- Focus on keeping the hips high throughout the movement. Before you start to pull the ball underneath, push the hips up and keep pushing. The line from your knees through your hips to your shoulders should be straight.

- Before removing the foot from the ball pause a second to focus on stabilizing. It will be tempting to allow your hip to drop when you take the foot off. Try not to.

- When straightening the leg keep the knees and thighs aligned with one another. This is a big step and the contraction in your hamstring is strong, so be prepared for this and make sure that you are properly warmed up.

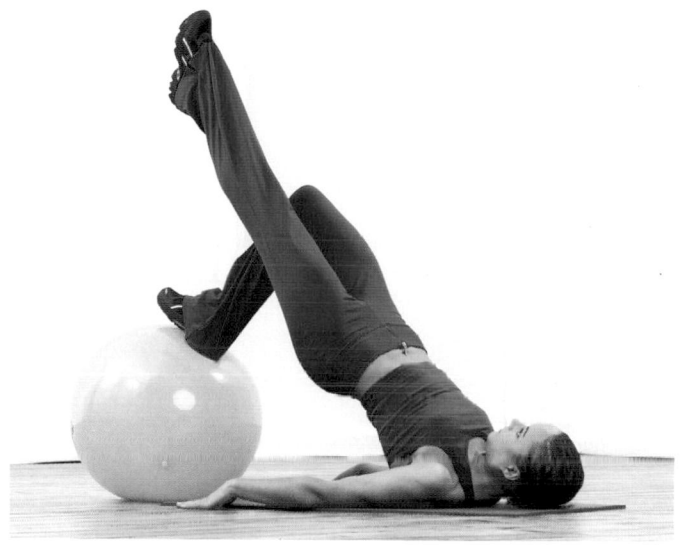

3 Lift one foot from the ball and straighten the leg. Replace your foot and roll the ball back out.

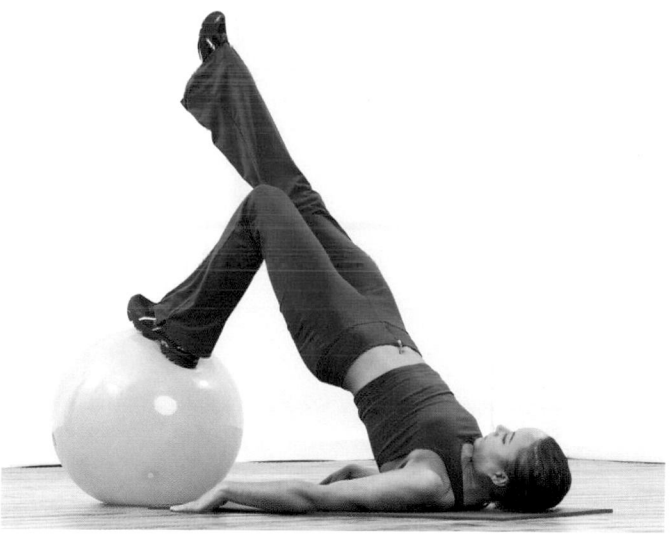

4 Pull the ball back in and lift the other foot from the ball, straightening the leg. Repeat this process, alternating the legs.

157

Glossary

Adaptation: The processes the body undergoes when responding to an increase in training and exercise.

Atrophy: The wastage of a muscle due to inactivity, illness, or age.

Base Metabolic Rate (BMR): The number of calories required for basic function during the day.

Cool-down: Exercises and stretching designed gradually to decrease the intensity of the workout and return the individual to a similar state as that of pre-exercise, in terms of heart rate and hormone levels. Also referred to as the "warm-down."

Concentric: The shortening of a muscle where the angle at a joint is decreased.

Delayed Onset Muscle Soreness (DOMS): Soreness felt in a muscle post-workout. Usually occurs within 24–48 hours. It is thought to be caused by the eccentric phase of the repetition producing microscopic tears in the muscle.

Dumbbell: Exercise tool made up of a short bar to fit in the hand and weight plates. Fixed versions have a non-variable weight.

Eccentric: The lengthening of a muscle where the angle at a joint is increased.

Flexibility: The maximum range of motion in a joint, or series of joints. There are three types: 1. Dynamic Flexibility: the ability to bring a limb through its full range of motion. 2. Static/Active Flexibility: the ability to assume and maintain an extended limb position using only your own muscles. 3. Static/Passive Flexibility: the ability to assume and maintain an extended limb position, using body weight, or a weight.

Heart Rate (HR): The number of times the heart beats in one minute (bpm).

Hypertrophy: An increase in the size of a muscle. This is thought to be due to an increase in the size of muscle fibers rather than the number of muscle fibers.

Intensity: The relative difficulty of an exercise as experienced by the individual. Reducing recovery time increases intensity.

Ligament: Connective tissue that joins bone to bone.

Maximum Strength: The greatest force that is possible in a single maximum muscle contraction.

Mobilize: Moving a joint through a range of movement to stimulate the release of synovial fluid, enabling the joint to move more freely.

Muscle: Tissue which crosses a joint to allow movement and made up of fibers. The muscle itself can only perform a pulling movement as it contracts and therefore muscles generally work in pairs to increase and decrease the angle of a joint.

Muscular Endurance: The ability of a muscle to perform a movement or a constant contraction for a number of repetitions, or a certain duration, before fatigue.

Overload: Applying a load which the body must overcome during exercise. This load is above what the body would normally lift.

Range of Movement (ROM): The full movement available at a joint. It is dependent on the health and shape of the joint itself and the flexibility of the attached muscle and connective tissue.

Repetition (rep): Moving a weight through a set range of movement once.

Resistance Tube/Band: A length of latex that, when stretched, creates a resistance to work against. They come in various tensions and styles.

Sets: A number of repetitions completed in succession. One set of 12 would mean doing 12 reps, one after another, before stopping.

Split Routine: Two or more workouts where different parts of the body are specifically targeted for training in each workout.

Strength Training: Activities that require the muscles to exert a force against some form of resistance. Also known as resistance training.

Superset: Two exercises done in quick succession with minimal rest in between. Traditionally done with opposing muscle groups.

Tendon: Connective tissue that joins muscle to bone.

Tri-Set: Three exercises completed in quick succession with minimal rest in between. Traditionally done with the same muscle group taken through three different types of movement.

Warm-up: A series of exercises designed to gradually elevate the heart rate, increase the core body temperature, and mobilize the joints.

Index

Acknowledgments

With thanks to our models Catherine and Philip, and photographer Eddie, for their patience. Thanks are due to my partner Sophie for the same reason. Thank you to my personal training clients who sacrificed their weekly hour of pain and pleasure so that I could concentrate on this book—though they need not worry, as I am sure I can make up for any discomfort they may have missed out on.

Mark Hatfield

Models: Philip Edelston, Catherine King
Photographer: Eddie Macdonald